Solutions for the Assessment of Bilinguals

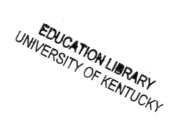

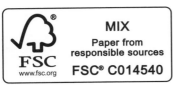
FSC
www.fsc.org

MIX
Paper from
responsible sources
FSC® C014540

Full details of all our publications can be found on http://www.multilingual matters.com, or by writing to Multilingual Matters, St Nicholas House, 31–34 High Street, Bristol BS1 2AW, UK.

Solutions for the Assessment of Bilinguals

Edited by
Virginia C. Mueller Gathercole

MULTILINGUAL MATTERS
Bristol • Buffalo • Toronto

Library of Congress Cataloging in Publication Data
Solutions for the Assessment of Bilinguals/Edited by Virginia C. Mueller Gathercole.
Includes bibliographical references and index.
1. Education, Bilingual—Ability testing. 2. Language arts—Ability testing. 3. Language and languages—Ability testing. 4. English language—Study and teaching—Foreign speakers. I. Mueller-Gathercole, Virginia C., editor of compilation.
LB1576.S66 2013
370.117'5–dc23 2013015534

British Library Cataloguing in Publication Data
A catalogue entry for this book is available from the British Library.

ISBN-13: 978-1-78309-014-3 (hbk)
ISBN-13: 978-1-78309-013-6 (pbk)

Multilingual Matters
UK: St Nicholas House, 31–34 High Street, Bristol BS1 2AW, UK.
USA: UTP, 2250 Military Road, Tonawanda, NY 14150, USA.
Canada: UTP, 5201 Dufferin Street, North York, Ontario M3H 5T8, Canada.

The policy of Multilingual Matters/Channel View Publications is to use papers that are natural, renewable and recyclable products, made from wood grown in sustainable forests. In the manufacturing process of our books, and to further support our policy, preference is given to printers that have FSC and PEFC Chain of Custody certification. The FSC and/or PEFC logos will appear on those books where full certification has been granted to the printer concerned.

Typeset by Techset Composition India (P) Ltd., Bangalore and Chennai, India.
Printed and bound in Great Britain by Short Run Press Ltd.

Contents

List of Tables and Figures

Tables

Figures

Contributors

Margareta Almgren Researcher; Member of ELEBILAB; UNESCO Chair on World Language Heritage
University of the Basque Country, San Sebastian/Donostia, Spain
Dr Almgren is a researcher in bilingualism, language acquisition and discourse.

Julia Barnes Lecturer in Language Learning and Teaching
Mondragon Unibertsitatea, Mondragón, Gipuzkoa, Spain
Dr Barnes is a researcher in the field of psycholinguistics with particular reference to early multilingualism in the home and at school.

Andoni Barreña Assistant Professor (Senior Lecturer) of Basque Linguistics; Member of ELEBILAB
Department of Spanish Linguistics, University of Salamanca, Salamanca, Spain; University of the Basque Country, San Sebastian/Donostia, Spain
Dr Barreña is a researcher in language acquisition (morphology, syntax, vocabulary) by early monolinguals and bilinguals, as well as in linguistic diversity.

Lisa M. Bedore Professor, Communication Sciences & Disorders
Department of Communication Sciences & Disorders, The University of Texas at Austin, Austin, TX, USA
Professor Bedore's research interests are in the areas of child language and phonological development and disorders, with a special interest in Spanish–English bilingual children. She is particularly interested in how aspects of language form – morphology and phonology in particular – interact with other aspects of language development.

Caroline Erdos Speech-Language Pathologist
Montreal Children's Hospital, Montreal, Quebec, Canada
Dr Erdos' expertise includes reading impairment, oral language impairment, bilingualism and multilingualism, cleft palate, attention deficit (+/– hyperactivity) disorder and foetal alcohol spectrum disorder.

María José Ezeizabarrena Senior Lecturer in General Linguistics; Member of ELEBILAB
Department of Linguistics and Basque Studies, University of the Basque Country, San Sebastian/Donostia, Spain
Dr Ezeizabarrena is a researcher in early language acquisition (morphology, syntax, vocabulary) in monolingual and bilingual settings.

Christine Fiestas Assistant Professor in Communication Sciences and Disorders; Speech-Language Pathologist
Department of Communication Sciences and Disorders, University of Hawai'i at Manoa, Honolulu, HI, USA
Dr Fiestas has research interests in the language and literacy acquisition of bilingual children, both with and without language impairment, and transfer of discourse skills across languages. She also works on using dynamic assessment techniques for non-biased testing of children from different language backgrounds.

Iñaki García Senior Lecturer in Data Analysis and Research Design: Non-experimental Method
Department of Social Psychology and Methodology of Behavioral Sciences (Faculty of Psychology), University of the Basque Country, San Sebastian/Donostia, Spain
Dr García has researched in the field of psycholinguistics and language acquisition.

Virginia C. Mueller Gathercole Professor of Linguistics (Miami, Florida) and Professor of Psychology (Bangor, Wales)
Linguistics Program, Florida International University, Miami, FL, USA; School of Psychology, Bangor University, Bangor, Wales, UK
Professor Gathercole has conducted research on monolingual and bilingual language acquisition in relation especially to semantics, morphosyntax and assessment. Her work also addresses issues concerning the relationship between language and cognition. She has specialized in Spanish–English, Welsh-English, and Spanish-Welsh bilinguals. She acted as Co-Director of the ESRC Centre for Research on Bilingualism in Theory and Practice, Bangor University, Wales, UK, from 2007 to 2012.

Fred Genesee Professor
Department of Psychology, McGill University, Montreal, Quebec, Canada
Professor Genesee's research interests focus on the achievement of students in alternative forms of bilingual education, simultaneous acquisition of two languages in pre-school children, the language development of internationally adopted children, and children at risk for reading and language impairment in a second language.

Kleanthes K. Grohmann Associate Professor of Biolinguistics
Department of English Studies, University of Cyprus and Cyprus Acquisition Team, Nicosia, Cyprus
A trained theoretical syntactician, Dr Grohmann founded the Cyprus Acquisition Team in order to systematically investigate language acquisition and development in Cyprus. The team looks at monolingual, bilectal and multilingual populations with typical as well as atypical and impaired language development, in particular SLI. He is the founding editor of the open-access journal *Biolinguistics* and the John Benjamins book series 'Language Faculty and Beyond'.

Corinne Haigh Assistant Professor
School of Education, Bishop's University, Lennoxville, Quebec, Canada
Dr Haigh's research focuses on literacy development in elementary school students in French Immersion programmes, with a particular emphasis on children at risk for difficulty with decoding and reading comprehension.

Erika Hoff Professor
Department of Psychology, Florida Atlantic University, Boca Raton, FL, USA
Dr Hoff's research focuses on bilingual development in the preschool period, on the role of input in bilingual development and on the sociocultural factors that shape children's dual language input.

Emma K. Hughes PhD Student
School of Psychology, Bangor University, Bangor, Wales, UK
Emma Hughes' PhD research focuses on bilingual aphasia, particularly cross-linguistic generalization of treatment effects in anomia.

Maria Kambanaros Associate Professor of Speech Pathology, Language Disorders and Multilingualism
Department of Rehabilitation Sciences, Cyprus University of Technology and Cyprus Acquisition Team, Nicosia, Cyprus
Dr Kambanaros is a certified bilingual speech pathologist with over 25 years of clinical experience and academic appointments in Greece and Cyprus. Her research interests are related to acquired and developmental language impairments in multilingual speakers, predominantly as related to the lexicon with an emphasis on assessment and treatment outcomes.

Carolyn Ann Letts Senior Lecturer
Speech & Language Sciences, School of Education, Communication and Language Sciences, Newcastle University, Newcastle Upon Tyne, UK
Dr Letts is a member of academic staff involved in teaching and research in speech and language impairment and the training of speech & language

therapists. Her particular interests include typical and impaired child language development, especially within a bilingual context, and the assessment of child language.

Ciara O'Toole Lecturer in Speech and Language Therapy
Department of Speech and Hearing Sciences, University College Cork, Cork, Ireland
Dr O'Toole's teaching and research interests are in the area of paediatric communication disorders, and bilingual language development in particular. She is currently developing assessment tools for children who are acquiring Irish in a bilingual context.

Elizabeth D. Peña Professor, Communication Sciences & Disorders; CCC-SLP
Department of Communication Sciences & Disorders, The University of Texas at Austin, Austin, TX, USA
Dr Peña studies the assessment and identification of bilingual children with and without language impairment. She focuses on ways to reduce bias in testing.

Rocío Pérez-Tattam Tutor in Spanish Language
Department of Spanish, Swansea University, Wales, UK
Dr Pérez-Tattam's research interests concern the interaction between the knowledge of two languages in the bilingual mind, differential language development in bilinguals compared to monolinguals, and issues of language assessment in bilinguals. She acted as a Postdoctoral Research Officer at the ESRC Centre for Research on Bilingualism in Theory and Practice, Bangor University, Wales, UK, from 2007 to 2012.

Eva Rodríguez-González Assistant Professor of Spanish Linguistics
Department of Spanish and Portuguese, Miami University, Oxford, OH, USA
Dr Rodríguez-González's research focuses on language processing, assessment of second language proficiency and second language acquisition research.

Robert Savage Associate Professor and William Dawson Scholar
Department of Education and Counselling Psychology, McGill University, Montreal, Quebec, Canada
Dr Savage's research focuses on the early development of reading and spelling strategies in typical and atypical learners. His research focuses on effective evidence-based intervention.

Hans Stadthagen-González Assistant Professor of Psychology (USM)
University of Southern Mississippi – Gulf Coast, Long Beach, MS, USA
Dr Stadthagen-González is a psycholinguist with two main fields of interest:
(1) language interaction in bilinguals at the interface between morphology
and syntax, and syntax and semantics; and (2) lexical processing in monolinguals and bilinguals, particularly concerning the variables that modulate
word recognition and production. He worked as a Postdoctoral Project
Researcher at the ESRC Centre for Research on Bilingualism in Theory and
Practice, Bangor University, Wales, UK, from 2007 to 2012.

Enlli Môn Thomas Senior Lecturer in Education
School of Education, Bangor University, Bangor, Wales, UK
Dr Thomas's main research interests span psycholinguistic studies of bilingual language acquisition, particularly in relation to children's acquisition of
complex structures under conditions of minimal input, and educational
approaches to language transmission, acquisition and use.

Feryal Yavas Senior Lecturer
Linguistics Program, Florida International University, Miami, FL, USA
Dr Yavas's research and teaching interests include language acquisition (first,
second and bilingual acquisition) and pragmatics/semantics.

1 Assessment of Bilinguals: Innovative Solutions

Virginia C. Mueller Gathercole

Volume 1 in this series, *Issues in the Asessment of Bilinguals,* contained a number of studies that argued for changes in the way in which bilingual children and adults are assessed, whether the assessment is of language itself or of cognitive and academic abilities that go beyond language. The authors provided evidence showing clearly that children growing up bilingually are not the same as children growing up monolingually and that even fully fluent bilingual adults perform distinctly from their monolingual peers. The authors in that volume argue that these differences pervade every area of the bilingual's linguistic knowledge – vocabulary, syntax, etc. – because of the linguistic and sociolinguistic experiences of bilinguals. The upshot of that work is that it is imperative to reformulate the ways in which we assess bilinguals.

The chapters in this volume – Volume 2 – take up this theme and propose some creative and innovative solutions to many of these issues. In some cases, researchers propose novel ways of testing children or adults in their second language (L2) to gain information on their abilities. In other cases, researchers propose ways of developing tools for assessing the first language (L1) of bilinguals and norming these for bilinguals. In other cases, the authors consider whether linguistic features shared by the bilingual's two languages (in the form of cognates) should be included or excluded from assessments. In still other cases the authors consider modifications to assessment that should take place in contexts in which either adequate information is not available regarding typical development in the L1 or in which changes occur in the patterns of input and, hence, the profiles observed, for bilinguals as they grow older.

We start with chapters that are concerned with the fact that assessment measures do not always exist for both of the languages that a child speaks. One cannot simply take a test developed for one language (e.g. English) and translate it to use for the other language. (This would be akin to testing a piano player with written music scripted for the drums or judging a hockey player's skating abilities on the basis of scoring criteria established for figure skaters.) These initial chapters examine how one could develop valid tests, either in the L2, or for an L1 for which no tests currently exist. The authors address the fact that the children or adults of concern are bilingual, and they discuss how this fact can affect the structure of the test itself or the participant's performance in particular aspects of the language.

In the first of these, 'Identification of Reading Difficulties in Students Schooled in a Second Language', Fred Genesee, Robert Savage, Caroline Erdos and Corrine Haigh center on the accurate identification of and effective intervention for L2-learning students with reading impairment in school. They specifically address the question of the best approach for assessing students for whom the school language is a second language. These authors provide a thoughtful and thorough review of the factors that might contribute to poor reading in L2 students. They stress that reading abilities may not just have to do with decoding, but with a range of other factors as well, including knowledge of the L2, knowledge of the cultural contexts of texts, and general cognition, including knowledge of the world and inferencing abilities.

They also provide a comprehensive picture of the research to date, suggesting that word-related, language-related and decoding skills relating to the child's L1 on entering school can be highly predictive of later reading abilities in the L2 and, hence, can provide early information to educators for the identification of which children may be in need of additional support or intervention. They argue, as a result, that one can test L2 children in their L1 (in Kindergarten) to obtain information on their decoding and language abilities (see also Burns, 2013), and this information can be used to predict reading decoding and reading comprehension of the L2 in Grades 1 and 3. In addition, their own data indicate that children may struggle with reading of the L2 for a variety of reasons – some children may have decoding-related difficulties, some may have language-related difficulties and some may have a combination of these. They suggest, therefore, that the best approach calls for assessment of the language abilities as well as the reading abilities of these children, in order to obtain a comprehensive profile of affected students' strengths and weaknesses. Some students might require intervention that focuses only on reading, while other students may need intervention that includes language as well as reading support.

While a great deal of the research on reading difficulties in children draws on a discrepancy model – wherein specific reading impairments are defined as involving reading difficulties in the absence of other (language, social, cognitive) difficulties – these researchers propose that a good alternative approach for such students is to use a dynamic approach, in which one observes a child's response to intervention (RtI). By monitoring a child's improvement over time, RtI can identify reading difficulties, regardless of the source of those difficulties. Such an approach allows for early intervention, in contrast to a 'wait-and-see' approach more typically related to a discrepancy model. By carefully monitoring a child's response to intervention, the practitioner can determine whether the child is progressing as might be expected or whether, instead, he or she needs further intervention. RtI allows early intervention and observation of children whose L1 may not be known by the practitioner. (One additional strength of such an approach is that it precludes having to 'label' students who are having difficulty as impaired or learning disabled – arguably one of the factors that contributes to practitioners' use of the 'wait-and-see' approach.)

In the next chapter, 'What are the Building Blocks for Language Acquisition? Underlying Principles of Assessment for Language Impairment in the Bilingual Context', Carolyn Letts turns to the issue of developing tests in a young child's L1 for the purpose of identifying language impairments (LI) in bilingual infants and toddlers. Letts discusses the fact that bilingual children's development in each of their languages looks different from development in monolinguals, so it is uninstructive, even inappropriate, to assess such children with tests that have been designed for monolinguals in just one of the languages. Children should be assessed in both their languages, but for many languages no tests are available, and we do not know much about normal developmental paths for those languages. Furthermore, we are still far from fully understanding how best to identify language impairments in bilingual children, whatever the language. The best way forward is complicated by a number of facts: (a) bilingual children's experience with language is very diverse, so it is difficult to draw inferences that apply to all of them; (b) we are lacking norms for bilingual development of language; (c) assessors, whether speech therapists or educational professionals, often lack knowledge of one or other of the child's languages; and (d) the linguistic performance of bilinguals in one or another of their languages might *look* quite similar to that of (monolingual) children with language impairment, but their profiles may look that way because of a lack of experience with the language in question, not due to an impairment (see, for example, Paradis, 2010, and commentaries).

Nevertheless, it is imperative to develop, when possible, assessment measures valid for each language in question, and in particular for bilinguals learning those languages. Letts touches on multiple key considerations that a test designer or language assessor needs to pay attention to, or that a speech language therapist (SLT) needs to be aware of, in order to assess bilingual children's potential language difficulties in any language. First, she emphasizes that, although we now know quite a bit about the likely 'markers' for linguistic impairment in English, we still need to discover what the nature of such markers might be for many of the distinct languages in question. What might be an area of difficulty for LI in one language (e.g. tense in English) might not be of relevance for LI in another language. Thus, we need tests designed for the specific languages of interest, based on the phenomena of relevance to the language in question, and preferably normed on bilingual children learning the language.

Second, as a first step towards developing such tests, we can take advantage of some key aspects of language development that appear to be universal – e.g. that one-word utterances evolve before multi-word utterances, that simple sentences emerge before complex sentences and that inferential skills and metalinguistic skills are generally late to emerge. Drawing on such universals, we can begin to search for guides as to how children pass through these stages in the language in question, keeping in mind that bilingual children may typically experience something of a lag in learning particular components of the language.

Third, Letts stresses that, while the possible markers of LI or of specific language impairment (SLI) will differ across languages, some commonalities we might be able to find as factors shared by language-impaired children of all backgrounds include the severity of the delay and difficulty in comprehension. She proposes possible vocabulary measures, elicitation of simple and complex sentences, and the use of spontaneous language samples in any tests developed.

In the following two chapters, work directed precisely at the development of such assessment measures for two particular languages is reported. These have to do with the development of versions of the CDI (Communicative Development Inventories) for two bilingual populations – first, Basque-speaking children, then Irish-speaking children. In both cases, the tests necessarily have to take into account the fact that children are growing up bilingually, since there are no children learning either language who are monolingual; all children learning both languages grow up as bilinguals.

In the case of Basque, María-José Ezeizabarrena, Julia Barnes, Iñaki García, Andoni Barreña and Margareta Almgren, in their chapter entitled 'Using Parental Report Assessment for Bilingual Preschoolers: The Basque Experience', discuss their efforts towards the development of a Basque CDI. Since Basque is a morphologically rich language, the CDI had to be adapted and structured to accommodate this richness. These researchers lay out in detail the steps they had to go through to develop a language-relevant version of the CDI for three age ranges, and they report on the general developmental trends for Basque. This includes information on the development of gestures, vocabulary comprehension, vocabulary production, morphology production and morphological complexity between 15 months and 50 months. Recognizing the fact that Basque-speaking children are usually bilingual or multilingual, the authors also discuss the performance of children with varying amounts of exposure to Basque. While differences are not so apparent early on (because of the paucity of data and the low level of performance at initial stages), differences by exposure appear more dramatic with age.

In the subsequent chapter, 'Using Parent Report to Assess Bilingual Vocabulary Acquisition: A Model from Irish', Ciara O'Toole proposes a novel way of dealing with the assessment of bilingual children in relation to Irish. While many people have taken a strategy of using two CDIs – one for each language– for children who speak two languages, in the case of Irish, given that most Irish-speaking children are growing up bilingually (in Irish and English), O'Toole has opted to develop a CDI for Irish that compiles information on both of the child's languages at the same time, in a single instrument. She proposes a bilingual version of the CDI that includes words common to Irish and English (i.e. loan words, cognates) entered as a single item, in contrast to words different in Irish and English, which are marked separately by the parent. She assesses the validity of the measure by comparing the information obtained from parents on this bilingual CDI (collected up to four times across two years per child) with information gleaned from spontaneous speech samples at the same collection points and finds a high correlation in the vocabulary knowledge they attribute to children.

O'Toole argues that the bilingual CDI constructed in this way streamlines the scoring process for parents, and parents do not have to 'decide' which language the common word represents. So far, Irish-dominant children have been tested with this measure. With further data, O'Toole plans to develop a version that will be normed according to the home language of the child – only Irish, Irish and English, and only English. This bilingual CDI can provide a good model for the assessment of other bilingual children across the globe.

In the next chapter, 'Development of Bilingual Semantic Norms: Can Two Be One?', Elizabeth D. Peña, Lisa M. Bedore and Christine Fiestas similarly focus on the unique challenges faced in relation to the assessment of bilingual children, especially if one wishes to distinguish language-impaired children from normally developing children. These authors focus on how one can develop tests to measure the bilingual child's proficiency in both languages in tandem. In order to develop parallel tests in the bilinguals' two languages, they argue, it is essential to follow well-tested psychometric principles. Using such principles, these researchers take us through the steps one can follow to develop such tests – in this case for Spanish–English bilinguals in Texas. They carefully discuss each step, from the choice of items for inclusion in the test to the development of norms that will serve to discriminate children with language impairment from normally developing bilinguals. In the choice of items, it is important to start from both languages ('dual focus') and to choose items that are not culturally skewed in favor of one population or the other. The items must also be sensitive to the traits of interest.

With pilot testing and careful analyses, Peña et al. show how one can design tests that are either linguistically equivalent across the two languages or psychometrically sensitive, depending on the goals for the use of the tests. A psychometrically sensitive test will include items that serve to maximally differentiate language-impaired from non-language impaired children, but at the same time yield minimal discrimination between children with different levels of language proficiency (e.g. Spanish-dominant, English-dominant, balanced) and experience. The principles set out by these authors can serve well as a guide for the development of similar valid measures for other bilingual populations.

Hans Stadthagen-González, Virginia C. Mueller Gathercole, Rocío Pérez-Tattam and Feryal Yavas turn to a different question in 'Vocabulary Assessment of Bilingual Adults: To Cognate or Not to Cognate'. They ask what elements can affect a bilingual's performance on assessments, and how it is best to approach those elements. They focus on 'external' factors, such as level of input, socio-economic factors and the like, as well as factors 'internal' to the languages in question and the relationship between them. They investigate the effects of these on performance in Spanish and English vocabulary tests by bilingual, end-state adults in Miami.

With regard to external factors, these authors found that, although all of the adults tested performed at or above the monolingual norm on the two tests, there was evidence of the influence of external factors on performance, such as which language(s) were spoken in the home when the participants were children, which language(s) they spoke in interaction with older siblings and friends, and the socio-economic level of their birth family.

Beyond these, an important question these authors address has to do with one 'internal' factor – lexical convergence between the two languages in cognates (or words that have similar forms and meanings in the two languages). Do bilinguals show better performance on cognates than on non-cognates in tests of vocabulary comprehension? Better performance would reveal cross-language facilitation either in acquiring these words or in processing these words in such tests.

The data from these adults indeed reveal superior performance in all bilingual groups on cognates over non-cognates. Further examination reveals that if one separates 'intuitive' cognates, or English words that even monolingual speakers of Spanish can 'guess' the meaning of, from others, the bilinguals perform even better on these than on non-cognates. These results are discussed in terms of their ramifications for the development of language tests for bilinguals and for our interpretation of such tests.

In Chapter 8, Maria Kambanaros and Kleanthes K. Grohmann face a somewhat different challenge. Their chapter, 'Profiling (Specific) Language Impairment in Bilingual Children: Preliminary Evidence from Cyprus', addresses assessment difficulties in relation to a community language for which adequate documentation regarding stages of development is lacking. In this case, the target language is Cypriot Greek, which is related to standard Greek, but whose status is debated – is it a separate dialect or a separate language from standard Greek? Regardless, this language variety varies considerably from standard Greek, so that materials available for standard Greek are inappropriate for use by language professionals and teachers wishing to conduct meaningful assessments of children's oral performance in Cypriot Greek. These authors discuss the development of materials for testing performance, and they report on two studies investigating knowledge of Cypriot

Greek in monolingual and bilingual typically developing children and children with SLI. In one study, they examine children's access to nouns and verbs; in the other, they look at children's performance in a story-telling task. In the latter, they pay particular attention to the amount of information provided, the number of subordinate clauses used and the length of the longest utterance.

When the performance of typically developing monolinguals, monolinguals with SLI and bilinguals with SLI is compared, these authors report that bilingual children with SLI perform in all respects like the monolingual children with SLI. They thus argue for a 'delayed' rather than 'deviant' approach for such children, and they conclude that the fact of having two (or more) languages does not lead to greater impairment in bilinguals than in monolinguals. They conclude with some implications of their work for language policy, language assessment and language treatment for bilingual children with SLI.

In the following chapter, it is not acquisition patterns related to a language for which normal patterns of development are unknown that is the issue, but acquisition patterns related to variations in the amount and types of input a child receives in a bilingual community, particularly in relation to the minority language. In 'Sociolinguistic Influences on the Linguistic Achievement of Bilinguals: Issues for the Assessment of Minority Language Competence', Enlli Môn Thomas, Virginia C. Mueller Gathercole and Emma K. Hughes explore the factors that influence the performance of Welsh-speaking children in Welsh. Previous research has shown that for both languages of Welsh–English bilinguals, the initial stages of development are directly linked to the amount of input children receive. Those who hear more English than Welsh perform better in English at early stages than those who hear more Welsh than English and those who hear Welsh and English equally, and those who hear more Welsh than English perform better at early stages in Welsh than those who hear more English than Welsh or who hear both languages about equally (Gathercole, 2010; Gathercole & Thomas, 2009). Furthermore, initial differences across groups tend to become neutralized with development and with the accumulation of some critical mass of input in the given language.

That neutralization is especially true for English, which can be attributed to the overwhelming presence and dominance of English in the community. For Welsh, the picture is more variable, and performance appears to be related to a variety of factors, including the language(s) spoken with peers, the domains of language use and the like.

An interesting pattern of development occurs with children who come from non-Welsh speaking homes: during the primary school years, their Welsh vocabulary knowledge, like that of their peers from Welsh-speaking homes, shows continual growth. This pattern changes, however, in the mid-teen years. At that point, the patterns of increases in Welsh vocabulary in this group depend on the prevalence of Welsh in their community. If they live in a community in which 65% or more of the population speaks Welsh, their vocabulary continues to improve. If, however, they live in a community with fewer than 65% Welsh speakers, their vocabulary appears to level off, with little or no improvement.

The implications for assessment, including the need to provide not only general age-determined norms of development but also home-language norms of development (as in Gathercole & Thomas, 2007), and possibly others, are discussed.

In one of the final chapters examining novel means of assessment, Eva Rodríguez-González is concerned with L2 acquisition (specifically Spanish as an L2) at the college level. In 'The Effects of Peer Feedback Practices in Spanish Second Language Writing', this author examines one strategy, peer feedback, that might be used to enhance L2 learners' literacy in that L2. She reports on a study in which L2 learners of Spanish were assigned to one of three treatment groups, one in which other students were trained for giving feedback on other students' written compositions, another in which untrained students gave feedback and a third (a control group) in which no such feedback was given. On examination of students' performance in the revisions of two compositions, a first one without students' feedback and a second one with the students' feedback, it appears that peer feedback was helpful in the revision process. The students in the group that received feedback from trained peers showed the most improvement in their rewriting of the second essay. In addition, students' responses on a written questionnaire showed that they generally found the peer feedback process a useful one. While they felt they could rely more on the instructor for feedback on the accuracy of their Spanish grammar, they were confident that their peers provided help on the content and organization of their essays. Rodríguez-González advocates further exploration of this method as a means to improving L2 teaching and at the same time keeping students engaged in the process.

In the final chapter, Erika Hoff reflects on the theoretical and practical import of the chapters in the two volumes. She provides an eloquent commentary on the importance of establishing norms for bilinguals, of determining appropriate measures and procedures, of attempting to provide measures that are equivalent across the bilingual's two languages, or across ages and domains, or across monolinguals and bilinguals, and of considering the impact of bilingualism on assessment in educational settings.

These chapters combined provide a resounding message regarding the assessment of bilingual children and adults. Although the challenges for finding appropriate solutions to the issues concerning the assessment of bilinguals are great, a variety of creative, innovative and thoughtful solutions will lead towards improved diagnoses, more accurate evaluation and a richer and more comprehensive picture of bilingual performance and abilities.

References

Burns, R. (2013) Assessment and instruction in multilingual classrooms. In V.C.M. Gathercole (ed.) *Issues in the Assessment of Bilinguals* (pp. 162–185). Bristol: Multilingual Matters.

Gathercole, V.C.M. (2010) Bilingual children: Language and assessment issues for educators. In K. Littleton, C. Wood and J. Kleine Staarman (eds) *Handbook of Psychology in Education* (pp. 713–748). Bingley: Emerald Group.

Gathercole, V.C.M. and Thomas, E.M. (2007) *Prawf Geirfa Cymraeg, Fersiwn 7–11*. [*Welsh Vocabulary Test, Version 7–11*]. Online at http://www.pgc.bangor.ac.uk

Gathercole, V.C.M. and Thomas, E.M. (2009) Bilingual first-language development: Dominant language takeover, threatened minority language take-up. *Bilingualism: Language and Cognition* 12, 213–237.

Paradis, J. (2010) The interface between bilingual development and specific language impairment. Keynote article for special issue with peer commentaries. *Applied Psycholinguistics* 31, 3–28.

2 Identification of Reading Difficulties in Students Schooled in a Second Language

Fred Genesee, Robert Savage, Caroline Erdos and Corrine Haigh

In this chapter, we discuss issues concerning the reading assessment of L2 students in general and of L2 students who are at risk of reading impairment in particular. We begin by defining reading impairment using the discrepancy view, a widely used definition, and discuss issues in the identification of students with reading impairment. We then review research findings that reveal both similarities and differences between L2 and L1 reading development that provide an empirical basis for planning reading assessment. This is followed by a discussion of a longitudinal study conducted in Montreal that was designed to examine the use of L1 abilities to predict individual differences in and risk for reading development in L2 students. This study also examined the extent to which reading and language difficulty overlap in L2 students. This study has a number of significant implications for the identification of at-risk L2 readers, issues that are discussed in detail in the next section of the chapter. In that section, we consider the advantages of a response-to-intervention approach, over the traditional discrepancy approach, to identifying at-risk L2 readers.

Oral and written language abilities play a crucial role in academic success. From the first day of school, learning is dependent on students' ability to understand and use oral language effectively for academic purposes. Beyond the primary grades, reading proficiency is essential for learning academic subject matter and new cognitive skills. Students with weak oral language and/or reading skills are at serious risk for academic failure and dropping out of school (Obadia & Thériault, 1997; Savage *et al.*, 2007; Snowling, 2000). In this chapter, we focus on students who struggle with learning to read, although we consider students who struggle with oral language development as well, especially insofar as there may be overlap in these two domains of language development. Our particular focus is on students being educated in a second language.

Many children around the world are educated through a second language (L2). For example, in countries where English is the dominant societal language (such as Canada, the United States and the United Kingdom), the proportion of non-English-speaking primary- and elementary-level students is substantial and may be 30% or more in some urban areas in these countries (e.g. DFES, 2010a; National Center for Educational Statistics, 2007). These students face a number of educational challenges in addition to learning English for the purposes of schooling, including adjustment to a new and sometimes unwelcoming culture, socializing into a new peer group, mastery of challenging academic knowledge and skills and, in some cases, overcoming trauma or difficulty related to immigration. Yet another group of L2 students is comprised of children who are educated in foreign or L2 immersion or bilingual school programs – such as English-speaking children in French or Spanish immersion programs in Canada and the United States, respectively, or English-speaking children in Welsh-medium schools in Wales. In contrast to the previous students who are members of minority language and culture groups, these L2 students are members of societally dominant groups and enjoy all of the privileges of majority group status. Yet other students who are educated in an L2 but are not immigrants are students from minority language groups who were born in the country in which they are being educated, such as children who speak aboriginal languages in South America and are educated in the official language of the country, for example, Spanish in Peru and Mexico. Often these children do not have access to education in their native language. The importance of reading is no less crucial for the academic success of L2 students than it is for students educated in their first language (L1).

The assessment of individual differences in students' reading abilities when they start school and periodically as they progress through school is critical for the purposes of instructional planning to ensure that all learners, be they L1 or L2, get the differentiated instruction they need to succeed in learning to read and ultimately in their schooling. Of particular concern in this chapter is assessment that is critical for the identification of L2 students who struggle with learning to read and thus require additional support. In some school districts, these students are eligible for supplementary services from reading specialists. The identification and provision of additional support for students with reading impairment may even be required by law in some areas.

In this chapter we discuss issues concerning the reading assessment of L2 students in general and of L2 students who are at risk of reading impairment in particular. We begin by defining reading impairment using the discrepancy view, a widely used definition, and discuss issues in the identification of students with reading impairment. We then review research findings that reveal both similarities and differences within L2 and L1 reading development which provide an empirical basis for planning reading assessment. This is followed by a discussion of a longitudinal study conducted in Montreal that was designed to examine the use of L1 abilities to predict individual differences in and risk for reading development in L2 students. This study also examined the extent to which reading and language difficulty overlap in L2 students. This study has a number of significant implications for the identification of at-risk L2 readers, issues that are discussed in detail in the next section of the chapter. In that section we consider the advantages of a response-to-intervention (RtI) approach, over the traditional discrepancy approach, to identifying at-risk L2 readers.

Defining Reading Impairment

According to the discrepancy model, one of the most widely used clinical definitions of reading impairment, students with reading impairment have great difficulty in learning to read accurately and fluently despite normal intelligence, normal visual-auditory abilities, adequate learning opportunities and the absence of neurological and psychological problems (see Savage & Deault, 2010, for a discussion of alternative definitions of reading impairment). This definition conceptualizes reading impairment as a developmental disorder that reflects underlying, probably genetically based, deficits in cognitive abilities and/or phonological processing that are linked specifically to reading in contrast to reading difficulties that are due to educational, medical, personal/social, socio-economic or other experiential factors. Diverse terms have been used to refer to reading impairment, including *dyslexia, specific developmental dyslexia* and *specific reading disability/impairment*. Definitions of reading impairment often focus on word-reading difficulties and, thus, refer to *dyslexia*. For example, the National Institute of Child Health and Human Development (NICHD, 2002) in the United States defined dyslexia as '... a specific language-based disorder of constitutional origin characterized by difficulties in single word decoding ...'.

While word reading is definitely the cornerstone of reading ability and often a major weakness in students with reading difficulties, there are reasons for adopting a conceptualization of reading difficulty that goes beyond decoding. Decoding alone cannot explain all the variance in reading ability among typical readers and, in particular, in individual differences in the comprehension of written text. One of the most influential theories of reading, the Simple View of Reading, recognizes listening comprehension along with decoding ability as a significant predictor of reading comprehension ability (Gough & Tunmer, 1986). Moreover, students who struggle with learning to read in either an L1 or an L2 can have difficulties with reading comprehension that do not include problems with decoding, difficulties that probably implicate higher order language skills, such as semantics or grammar (Bishop & Snowling, 2004; Catts et al., 2005; Erdos et al., 2011); these students are sometimes referred to as 'poor comprehenders' (Bishop & Snowling, 2004; see Catts et al., 2005, for an alternative view). It has been estimated that 5–10% of English-speaking school children in the United States display this reading profile (Catts et al., 2005; Nation, 2005). While the precise difficulties of 'poor comprehenders' are not yet well understood, it is thought that some of these struggling readers may have language impairment that either has gone undetected and untreated or is not sufficiently severe to fall within clinically defined definitions. In these cases, it may be that it is their language impairment that is responsible for their reading comprehension difficulties.

As yet, there is no reliable estimate of the extent of co-occurrence of reading and language impairment. This is an important practical as well as theoretical issue. If the evidence indicates high rates of overlap, this could imply that reading and language impairment are different manifestations of the same underlying disorder; low prevalence of overlap would imply different or distinct impairments. In either case, accurate identification of and effective intervention for students with reading impairment calls for assessment of their language abilities as well as their reading abilities in order to obtain a comprehensive profile of affected students' strengths and weaknesses. This, in turn, is needed in order to maximize intervention gains and reduce the number of students who develop chronic difficulties (e.g. Scanlon et al., 2008a, 2008b; Wallach, 2007).

Rates of Reading Impairment

It has been estimated that as many as 20% of the school-age population in the United States may be affected by a reading impairment (Shaywitz & Shaywitz, 2005). Similarly high rates of difficulty in acquiring grade-appropriate levels of reading ability have been reported in other countries (DFES, 2010b; Statistics Canada, 2004; Willms & Murray, 2007). There are no statistics that we know of that estimate the prevalence of reading impairment in L2 students. Despite the lack of reliable statistics, there is no reason to believe that rates of reading (or language) impairment should be higher in L2 learners than among monolingual school-age children. Evidence that bilingual or L2 status alone is not a risk factor comes from studies in Canada which have not shown elevated rates of reading difficulty among non-English-speaking immigrant students in comparison to native English-speaking students. In fact, immigrant L2 learners in this country often score as well as or better than native-born students on tests of reading achievement in secondary school and have equal or better rates of secondary school graduation (Garnett, 2006; OECD, 2006). Evaluations of the academic achievements – including reading achievements – of both minority-language and majority-language students who participate in bilingual school programs in the United States and Canada, respectively, have found that they score as well as their peers in monolingual programs on a variety of reading tests, indicating further that L2 status alone is not a risk factor for reading impairment (Genesee, 2007; Genesee & Lindholm-Leary, 2012). Similarly, there is no reason to believe that risk for language impairment is linked to bilingualism or L2 learning (Gutiérrez-Clellen et al., 2008; Paradis et al., 2003; see Chapter 9 in Paradis et al., 2011, for a review). Both Paradis et al. and Gutiérrez-Clellen and colleagues found that bilingual children (primarily simultaneous bilinguals) who had been diagnosed with specific language impairment exhibited the same patterns and degree of impairment as children with language impairment who were learning the same languages monolingually (namely, French and English for Paradis, and Spanish and English for Gutiérrez-Clellen).

Although not at greater risk for reading impairment, L2 students may be at greater risk for reading difficulties of a non-clinical nature. For example, it has been estimated that as many as two out of every three Grade 4 Spanish-speaking English language learners in the United States are unable to read English at a level that is sufficient to support their success in school (August & Hakuta, 1998; Sanchez et al., 2004). L2 students may be more likely to struggle with learning to read for a variety of reasons, including, for example, interrupted or inappropriate schooling, poverty, inadequate medical attention, socio-economic factors in the home, or other experiential factors. In light of the high probability that many L2 students might experience difficulty in learning to read, an approach to identification and intervention that includes these struggling L2 readers is recommended. We return to this issue in the section on 'Identification of Struggling L2 Readers'.

Issues in the Identification of Reading Impairment

Identification of students with reading impairment following the discrepancy definition discussed earlier entails comprehensive assessment of students' intellectual, perceptuo-motor and neurocognitive abilities, along with their reading abilities. The former are tested in order to determine if the student's reading difficulties are due to reading-specific deficits or to other experiential or developmental issues. Thus, the identification of students with or at risk for reading impairment is a complicated matter because it involves both inclusionary and exclusionary factors; moreover, the assessment of each can be problematic. Inclusionary factors include performance on reading-related tests or tasks that is substantially below the norm, often taken to be at least 1 or 1.5 standard deviations below the mean of the norming group. Lesaux and Geva *et al.* (2008: 50) note that the most common criterion for identifying reading impairment in studies of English language learners in the United States is a score on a standardized reading test at or below the 25th percentile. While lower-than-expected levels of reading performance provide primary evidence that an individual student is struggling with learning to read, this alone is not sufficient to identify the source of the difficulty and, specifically, whether his or her low performance reflects an underlying impairment that is specific to reading.

Exclusionary factors must also be considered in order to rule out other conditions and factors that might explain students' reading difficulties. In the case of L1 students, exclusionary factors include: visual, auditory or other sensorimotor problems; below average intelligence; frank neurological disorders; no or inadequate prior experiences with reading (such as poor instruction in school); and social and/or personal issues. If a struggling reader's difficulties appear to be linked to one or a number of these factors, then specific reading impairment is less probable. These exclusionary factors also apply to the identification of impairment in struggling L2 readers. An additional important exclusionary factor in the case of L2 students is incomplete acquisition of the target language that prevents students from reading at grade- or age-appropriate levels. It can be difficult to disentangle opportunity to learn the L2 from reading impairment, especially when L2 learners first begin schooling in the L2 and have had insufficient time to learn the language. The assessment of exclusionary factors does not entail only formal testing and often includes careful and thorough collection of information about students' histories using structured interviews or questionnaires. Collecting information about exclusionary factors can be difficult if students and/or their parents do not speak the L2 well. In the absence of school personnel who speak the parents' language, an interpreter or cultural broker in the community who speaks the student's home language and is familiar with the home culture may be required to collect this information.

Although research indicates that students who struggle with learning to read benefit from early systematic intervention (Gersten & Geva, 2003; Lesaux & Siegel, 2003; Mathes *et al.*, 2007; Vaughn *et al.*, 2006), educators often take a 'wait-and-see' approach to identifying at-risk L2 readers on the assumption that their reading difficulties are due to incomplete acquisition of the L2 and, thus, will resolve once they have been in school longer. While this may be true for some struggling L2 students, it is not likely for many and especially for L2 learners with reading impairment. Delaying intervention for these L2 readers can result in chronic literacy and academic problems later on, even among students with reading difficulties of a non-clinical nature. Many problems can be avoided, or at least minimized, if appropriate classroom intervention is provided early (e.g. Al Otaiba *et al.*, 2009). Thus, there are shortcomings in this method of identification of reading impairment, and we return to these in the section on 'Identification of Struggling L2 Readers'.

Understanding Reading Acquisition

The identification of students with reading difficulties and/or impairment requires an understanding of L2 reading acquisition in order to distinguish typical from atypical patterns and rates of development in individual students. Similarly, the provision of appropriate and effective support for students who are struggling with learning to read, for clinical or non-clinical reasons, requires an understanding of the possible sources of difficulty that individual students are facing. While a great deal of research on L1 reading acquisition is available to guide assessment and intervention, there is much less on L2 reading acquisition, and most of this has focused on students who begin their schooling in the L2 in the primary grades. Nevertheless, there is currently sufficient evidence to inform assessment policies and practices, keeping in mind that the picture will change as more evidence emerges. In this section, we briefly review current evidence on reading acquisition among elementary school-age students that is relevant to reading assessment and intervention. We reference research on both L2 and L1 students, and we focus on evidence pointing to important similarities and differences in L2 and L1 reading acquisition. Examining evidence of similarities between L2 and L1 readers is useful since it can indicate to what extent knowledge linked to L1 reading development is relevant to assessment and intervention for struggling L2 readers. At the same time, understanding differences in L2 and L1 reading is critical to respond to the specific needs of L2 readers.

Similarities in L2 and L1 reading development

The extensive and ever-expanding body of research on L1 reading acquisition and the growing body of research on L2 reading acquisition indicate some fundamental similarities in L1 and L2 reading acquisition that are useful for the identification of at-risk L2 readers. In general, the evidence from both sources paints a picture of a process that is multi-componential, hierarchical and developmental in nature. First of all, reading acquisition is multi-componential because it involves diverse interrelated skills and knowledge and, more specifically, phonological awareness (PA), letter-sound knowledge, vocabulary and knowledge of complex grammar. In addition, and arguably just as importantly, learning to read entails sustained motivation and interest and certain background knowledge. Some of these skills and knowledge are linked specifically to processing written language, such as PA and letter-sound knowledge; some are related to general language competence – for example, knowledge of how verb tense, pronouns and connectors are used to create a timeline in narratives; yet others entail general or world knowledge and, thus, are not language specific at all. For the purposes of this chapter, we focus on language-related skills and knowledge because they are particularly useful for assessment purposes, but it is important to emphasize that learning to read entails other kinds of skills, knowledge and predispositions.

Second, and with respect to the language-related skills and knowledge that underpin reading, learning to read entails both 'word-level' and 'text-level' skills. Word-level skills include knowledge of the letters of the alphabet and of letter clusters and their commonly associated sounds (phonemes), PA and word decoding itself (i.e. blending phonemes to assemble word pronunciations). Other word-level knowledge, including word-specific orthographic knowledge, is also required for the many words that are exceptions to spelling rules in opaque orthographies such as English and French (Share, 2008). Together these phonological and orthographic skills, along with word-specific semantic skills, underlie word-level reading skills in English as an L1 (Bishop & Snowling, 2004; Castles & Nation, 2006; Share, 2008). There is growing, albeit incomplete, evidence that these kinds of skills and knowledge similarly underlie word-level reading skills in English as an L2 (August & Shanahan, 2006; Riches & Genesee, 2006; Share, 2008).

Text-level skills go beyond reading isolated words and involve skills and knowledge implicated in comprehending written and oral sentences and text/discourse, such as knowledge of complex grammar and narrative structure. While word-level skills are modular insofar as they can develop in isolation of text-level skills, text-level skills necessarily entail word-level along with sentence-level and more general language and cognitive skills, as noted earlier. In this sense then, the major linguistic units that underpin reading development can be said to be hierarchically organized (e.g. Perfetti, 2003, 2007; Shatil & Share, 2003).

Finally, reading acquisition, like the acquisition of many skills and knowledge in school, is cumulative or developmental in nature. To be more specific, certain skills and knowledge, like PA, phonics (learning to map sounds onto letters) and decoding, serve as building blocks for acquiring higher order reading skills linked to comprehension of written text. Failure to acquire competent word-level skills and knowledge can impede the acquisition of text-level comprehension skills. Moreover, word-level skills must be acquired to a high level of competence so that cognitive resources can be devoted to comprehending complex text (Perfetti, 2003, 2007).

The results from research on L1 and L2 reading acquisition indicate that learning to read in an L2 is like learning to read in an L1 in even more specific ways that can guide the assessment of L2 students for purposes of identifying those who are at risk for reading difficulty (e.g. Erdos *et al.*, 2011; see also

August & Shanahan, 2006; Genesee & Jared, 2008; Genesee *et al.*, 2006, for reviews). First, predictors of word-decoding ability in L1 students are also significant predictors of word-decoding ability in L2 students. For example, phonological processing, and PA in particular, along with knowledge of letter-sound relationships in English, have been found to be the most consistently significant, although not the only, predictors of word-decoding skills in English as a second language as in English as a first language. This is true for both minority-language students (August & Shanahan, 2006; Lesaux & Geva *et al.*, 2008; Riches & Genesee, 2006) and majority-language group students (Erdos *et al.*, 2011; Genesee & Jared, 2008). Of additional importance, these predictors are significant crosslinguistically as well as intralinguistically so that individual variation in phonological processing (particularly PA) and letter-sound knowledge in the L1 correlates with variation in ability in the corresponding skills in the L2 and with individual variation in L2 word-decoding ability (Genesee & Geva, 2006; Geva & Clifton, 1994; Jared *et al.*, 2011). Thus, assessment of L2 students' knowledge and ability in these domains in the L1 could be used as proxies for assessing their ability in these domains in L2 when they have insufficient competence in the L2 for L2 assessments to be valid. The significance of this for identification will be discussed later.

The precise 'grain' of phonological processing that overlaps in biliteracy development may be even more specific. In closely related languages, such as English and French, it appears that ability with respect to processing specific types of phonological units in students' L1 predicts acquisition of reading in L2. More specifically, Haigh *et al.* (2011) investigated the links between phoneme awareness and onset-rime awareness with reading outcomes in native English-speaking students who were being educated and learning to read in French as a second language. Both a phoneme manipulation task and a closely matched vowel-consonant phoneme and consonant-vowel onset-rime awareness task (e.g. 'ea-t' and 't-ea') were administered to 98 children in English and French in the spring of their Kindergarten (K) year. Regression analyses indicated that English phoneme manipulation was a significant predictor of both English and French reading outcomes at the end of Grade 2, after controlling for knowledge of letter names and word identification skills in K. In contrast, English onset-rime manipulation was a weak predictor. French onset-rime knowledge in K accounted for significant variance in French reading outcome measures only. These results thus support the existence of a link between English phoneme manipulation in K and both English and French reading outcomes in Grade 2. Practically speaking, these results provide important assessment information about what kind or 'grain' of PA measures can be used in K to predict later reading outcomes for children learning to read in an L2.

In theoretical terms, these results are important because they do not fit well with theories such as Ziegler and Goswami's (2005) influential

Psycholinguistic Grain Size (PGS) hypothesis. The PGS hypothesis predicts orthography-specific effects of rimes and phonemes on acquisition, wherein rimes should have a stronger impact on reading in opaque orthographies such as English (which has many exceptions to grapheme-to-phoneme correspondence rules) than they do in more transparent orthographies (where such rules always or often produce accurate pronunciations of words). French is not entirely transparent for reading but is much more so than English. On the basis of the PGS hypothesis, therefore, one might have expected a greater role for phonemes in French than in English, and vice versa for rimes; however, our results did not find this.

L2 and L1 reading acquisition are also similar with respect to certain aspects of reading comprehension, although there is much less research on reading comprehension than on decoding. Current evidence indicates that L2 and L1 reading comprehension are similar at a very general level insofar as a variety of individual difference and contextual factors may play important roles. More specifically, and importantly from an assessment point of view, language-related factors that influence the acquisition of L2 reading comprehension, as they do L1 reading comprehension, include word decoding, vocabulary, oral proficiency and listening comprehension skills in the language being read (Lesaux & Geva et al., 2008; Riches & Genesee, 2006). The precise ways in which these language-related skills influence comprehension in L2 and L1 students are still questions that require empirical investigation.

There has been little research examining L2 students with reading impairment per se. As a result, for the most part, we can only infer from findings about individual differences in L2 reading development what the results for L2 students with impairment would be like. Extant research shows that minority- and majority-language L2 students who experience difficulty in learning to decode demonstrate weaknesses in PA and in their knowledge of letter-sound relationships (e.g. Erdos et al., in press; Genesee & Jared, 2008; Lesaux & Geva et al., 2008). This is not surprising, given the results from the research on individual differences in word decoding reviewed earlier. L2 students, again from both majority and minority groups, with poor reading comprehension skills, like their L1 counterparts, often have poor decoding skills along with poor language skills related to vocabulary, listening comprehension and morphosyntax (August & Shanahan, 2006; Lesaux & Kieffer, 2010; Lesaux et al., 2010; Riches & Genesee, 2006). However, the specific pattern of weaknesses in language that are associated with comprehension difficulties may depend on the students' grade level. More specifically, weaknesses in word decoding are more likely to be significant correlates of comprehension difficulty during relatively early stages of reading development, to the extent that young readers adopt a word-by-word approach to reading text. In contrast, complex language skills are likely to become important as students progress through school and confront increasingly complex texts. Studies of reading comprehension in L1 students in Grade 5 and above suggest that even higher order skills, such as inference-making ability, comprehension monitoring and sensitivity to story structure, may play significant roles when reading advanced-level texts (Muter *et al.*, 2004; Oakhill *et al.*, 2003). It would not be surprising if this were the case for L2 students as well. Thus, assessment of struggling L2 readers in later stages of development should include both word-level and language-related abilities in order to pinpoint the nature of their difficulties.

It is important also to recognize that variation in the correlates of reading comprehension may reflect variation in what specific tests assess. More specifically, it has been found that some reading comprehension tests reflect variation in performance that is due largely to decoding ability and relatively little else (Lesaux *et al.*, 2010; Nation & Snowling, 1997). In other words, comprehension of the text in these tests relies relatively little on higher level language skills. In addition, some comprehension tests may assess general knowledge rather than the ability to extract knowledge from the text itself (e.g. Keenan & Betjemann, 2006). This is a particularly important issue to consider when assessing L2 students whose general knowledge is often different from that of mainstream students. Thus, it is important to consider the quality of available tests, especially reading comprehension tests, when interpreting L2 students' test results.

Differences in L2 and L1 reading development

Notwithstanding these important similarities between L2 and L1 reading acquisition, there are also important differences that must be considered during assessment and intervention. L2 students differ from L1 students with respect to reading development in a number of important ways: (1) L2 students often have different cultural orientations, world knowledge and social experiences, or what Moll and colleagues refer to as 'funds of knowledge' (Gonzalez *et al.*, 2005); (2) they know and use another language – their L1; and (3) L2 students are still learning the L2. All three factors can influence the way in which L2 students learn to read and, as well, the speed, fluency and accuracy with which they read. These, in turn, can result in differences in test performance that could be misinterpreted as evidence of reading impairment or difficulty.

First, educational materials and instructional approaches – and, importantly, reading texts – are often based on the cultural backgrounds of majority language students. It is usually relatively easy for majority language students to understand and relate to the content of what they are reading and being taught, especially in the early grades. But for minority language L2 students, differences in cultural background can make it difficult to comprehend such materials or to perform well on the standardized reading tests used to screen for reading difficulty or impairment (Genesee & Geva, 2006;

Geva & Clifton, 1994; Jared et al., 2011; Riches & Genesee, 2006). Practically speaking, it is important, therefore, to use assessment materials and tasks with content familiar to L2 students. Tests should focus on reading ability, not on the understanding of unfamiliar material or procedures.

Second, L2 reading acquisition also differs from L1 reading acquisition because L2 students know another language (their L1), and research has shown that they often draw on knowledge about and skills in their L1 when reading in the L2 (August & Shanahan, 2006; Genesee & Geva, 2006; Riches & Genesee, 2006). Using the L1 to scaffold reading in the L2 is most useful during the early stages of reading acquisition when students have not fully acquired the L2. In this stage, L2 students may draw on word-level skills in the L1 to decode words in the L2. Using the L1 to scaffold L2 reading can also be useful even later when students are expected to read more advanced text. At these later stages, L2 students may transfer strategies for figuring out the meanings of unfamiliar words or for monitoring comprehension of what they are reading, for example (Riches & Genesee, 2006); the more similar the L1 and L2 (as is the case for Spanish and English in comparison to Mandarin and English, for example), the greater the transfer (Bialystok et al., 2005). If students transfer specific skills and strategies from the L1 when reading in the L2 and this produces the correct response in the L2, the influence of the L1 is invisible. In these cases, we simply think that they 'got it right'. It is transfer from the L1 resulting in errors in the L2 that is noticed. Because most transfer effects that are noticed are linked to errors in the target language, it has often been thought that L2 learners should keep their L1 and L2 separate. In some schools, L2 learners have even been punished for using the L1 on this assumption. However, rather than interpreting transfer errors as signs of incompetence, it is more appropriate to interpret them as students' active attempts to fill in gaps in their L2 by drawing on corresponding skills and knowledge from the L1 – a kind of linguistic bootstrapping (Genesee et al., 2006). Interpretation of transfer errors as deficiencies in L2 learners' reading abilities can contribute to overestimates of reading difficulty in L2 learners.

Third, and finally, L2 learners obviously differ from students learning to read in their L1 because they are still learning the L2. In particular, they are still acquiring advanced level morphosyntactic and discourse skills of the type that are likely to underpin comprehension of advanced written texts (e.g. Deacon et al., 2007; see August & Shanahan, 2006, for a review of research on this topic). From an assessment point of view, these findings indicate that it is important always to assess within L2 students' proficiency limits so that the test functions as a reading test and not a test of language competence. This is especially true when assessing L2 students in the early stages of L2 reading development. This also means that intervention for struggling L2 readers should include oral language development along with a focus on reading-specific skills.

The Montreal At Risk Reading Study

Our own longitudinal research on the reading development of L2 students in Montreal illustrates that L1 test results can be useful in predicting both individual differences in and risk for reading difficulty in an L2 (see Erdos *et al.*, 2011, in press). In this study, we examined predictors of reading ability in French as a second language in a group of 86 English-speaking children who were participating in an early total French immersion program. All instruction, including reading, in this program was in French, the students' L2, during K and Grade 1. English was introduced as a language of instruction in Grade 2 and gradually increased thereafter to include about 50% of instructional time. A battery of tests was administered to the students in K which were used to predict their subsequent word-decoding and reading comprehension abilities in French at the end of Grades 1, 2 and 3. We also included predictor and achievement tests of their language abilities in order to ascertain to what extent language difficulties are a concomitant problem for children at risk for reading difficulties, as has been hypothesized by some (e.g. Bishop & Snowling, 2004). Table 2.1 includes a list of the tests used in the study. The predictor battery included tests that have been shown by previous research to be significantly related to individual differences, including risk for impairment, in either reading or language development in English as a first language (see Erdos *et al.*, in press, for more details). These included, for example, a blending task, in which the children were orally presented with two or three isolated syllables comprised of a consonant followed by a vowel (CV: 't-ea'), a vowel followed by a consonant (VC: 'ea-t'),

Table 2.1 Fall/spring Kindergarten predictors

Reading related

Phonological awareness (blending)[a]
Letter-sound knowledge
Letter-name knowledge [b]
Word decoding [b]

Language related

Receptive vocabulary – English, French [c,d]
Expressive morphology [e]
Sentence recall [f]

[a] Comaskey *et al.* (2009).
[b] Wide Range Achievement Test 3: Blue Reading Subtest (Wilkinson, 1993).
[c] Peabody Picture Vocabulary Test (Dunn & Dunn, 1997).
[d] Échelle de vocabulaire en images Peabody (Dunn *et al.*, 1993).
[e] Test of Early Grammatical Impairment (Rice & Wexler, 2001).
[f] Clinical Evaluation of Language Fundamentals 4 (Semel *et al.*, 2003)

or a consonant followed by a vowel and a consonant (CVC: 'b-ea-t'), and were asked to put them together (i.e. blend) to make a word. There were nine CV, nine VC and nine CVC items in total. The predictor tests were administered in the students' L1 in order to determine: (1) if and to what extent they could predict individual differences in the students' subsequent L2 reading and language abilities; and (2) to what extent they could predict risk for L2 reading and/or language impairment. A test of French receptive vocabulary (*Échelle de vocabulaire en images Peabody* (EVIP); Dunn *et al.*, 1993) was also administered in K to determine to what extent prior knowledge of French predicted later reading scores in French. The predictor tests were administered in both the fall and spring of K, their first year of schooling, in order to determine how early we could predict risk for later L2 reading and language difficulties. French reading comprehension outcome scores were based on a combination of scores on both the word and sentence comprehension subtests of the BEMEL (Cormier *et al.*, 2006). Listening comprehension was assessed in English using the Sentence Structure subtest of the Clinical Evaluation of Language Fundamentals-4 (CELF-4; Semel *et al.*, 2003) and, in French, using a French version of this test (see Erdos *et al.*, in press, for more details). Because of space limitation, we focus on the Fall-K predictors.

Predicting individual differences

Two sets of regression analyses were run to examine the extent to which the Fall-K test results could predict individual differences in L2 reading achievement, both word reading and reading comprehension, at the end of Grade 1 and again at the end of Grade 3. With respect to word decoding in French at the end of Grade 1, two significant predictors emerged: letter-name knowledge in English and receptive vocabulary in French. These two predictors accounted for 24% of the variance in the Grade 1 word-decoding scores. With respect to Grade 3 decoding in French, blending in English and receptive vocabulary in French emerged as significant predictors and accounted for 20% of the variance.

With respect to reading comprehension in French at the end of Grade 1, both letter-name knowledge in English and English blending emerged as significant predictors, implying that decoding-related skills in English were significantly related to subsequent reading comprehension abilities in the students' L2. French receptive vocabulary was also a significant predictor along with performance on the rapid automatized naming (RAN) of familiar objects in English. Performance on RAN-objects has been associated with general language abilities (and deficits) (e.g. Catts *et al.*, 2002). Together, these four predictors accounted for 55% of the variance in the Grade 1 reading comprehension scores in French.

Significant predictors of Grade 3 reading comprehension results included a combination of word-level predictors (namely, letter-name knowledge in

English) and language-related predictors (namely, English and French receptive vocabulary and RAN-objects in English). Together, these four predictors accounted for 42% of the variance in the Grade 3 reading comprehension scores. Predictions of the Grade 3 outcomes are noteworthy given the lag between the predictor test results and the outcome results. The fact that both word-related and language-related skills emerged as significant predictors of reading comprehension supports previous findings that reading comprehension is dependent on both – a theory espoused by the Simple View of Reading (Hoover & Gough, 1990).

The simple view of L2 reading

Further evidence of the importance of both word-decoding and language-related skills for the development of reading comprehension skills in an L2 emerged in the statistical analyses we conducted to examine the Simple View of Reading. Briefly, according to the Simple View, reading comprehension (RC) is the result of the product of decoding (D) and listening comprehension (LC) abilities, and not their simple additive effects. That is, $RC = D \times LC$ (Hoover & Gough, 1990). While there has been considerable support for the Simple View of Reading (Gough & Tunmer, 1986; Hoover & Gough, 1990; Joshi & Aaron, 2000), some researchers have been unable to replicate the multiplicative effect proposed by this view with English-L1 learners (Chen & Vellutino, 1997; Kirby & Savage, 2008; Savage, 2006; Savage & Wolforth, 2007). We examined the validity of the Simple View both intra-linguistically and crosslinguistically using regression analyses; that is to say, in one set of analyses, we included French-L2 predictors and French-L2 reading comprehension outcomes and, in another set of analyses, we used English-L1 predictors and French-L2 outcomes. In contrast to the previous regression analyses which used scores from K to predict individual differences in Grade 1 and 3 reading outcomes, these regression analyses were run using predictor scores from the end of Grade 1 along with outcome measures also from the end of Grade 1. Concurrent Grade 1 predictors were analyzed because the Simple View is a hypothesis about concurrent correlates of reading comprehension. In our analyses, additive as well as multiplicative effects of decoding and listening comprehension were entered as separate predictors.

While we failed to find crosslinguistic evidence in support of the model, there was statistically significant support for it intra-linguistically. To be more specific, our analyses revealed that Grade 1 French pseudo-word decoding was a highly significant concurrent predictor of reading comprehension ($ß = 0.725, p < 0.001$), whereas Grade 1 French listening comprehension alone was not. The analyses also revealed that there was a significant interaction between French pseudo-word decoding and listening comprehension ($ß = -0.262, p = 0.001$). Together, these predictors accounted for over half of the variance in the Grade 1 French reading comprehension test scores: ($R^2 = 0.553$), $F(2,83) = 51.364$, $p < 0.001$. Analysis of the interaction effect indicated that students with good decoding skills scored higher overall and that, although good listening comprehension skills enhanced the reading comprehension scores of students with good decoding skills, they provided little advantage for students with poor decoding skills. In short, the benefit of good listening comprehension skills was contingent on students' decoding abilities.

Predicting risk for L2 reading difficulties

We subsequently conducted discriminant analyses to see if the K predictors in English could discriminate between students who were considered at risk at the end of Grade 1 for reading difficulties in their L2 and students who were not (see Erdos *et al.*, in press, for more details). We also explored the extent to which risk for reading and language difficulty in an L2 are distinct or overlapping risks. In order to do this, we identified Grade 1 students who were at risk for L2 reading difficulties and, independently, students who were at risk for L2 language difficulties. In fact, we identified two at-risk reading groups, one at risk for word decoding in L2 and one at risk for reading comprehension in their L2. A student was considered 'at risk' for decoding if, at the end of Grade 1, he or she scored more than one standard deviation below the mean of the entire sample on the French pseudo-word decoding subtest of the Wechsler Individual Achievement Test (2nd edition), original French-Canadian Version (Wechsler, 2005). Students were considered 'not at risk' if they scored within one standard deviation of the group mean on this test. Risk for reading comprehension was determined using student performance on the Grade 1 word comprehension and sentence comprehension subtests of the BEMEL (Cormier *et al.*, 2006, original French version). The at-risk and not-at-risk language subgroups were similarly identified. In this case, risk was based on performance on both the Concepts and Following Directions and the Sentence Structure subtests of the CELF-4 (Semel *et al.*, 2003), administered in English in the spring of Grade 1.

In order to reduce the number of predictor measures in these analyses, we conducted principal components analysis of all K predictor test scores (both reading- and language-related). This was done using both fall and spring predictor results, but for sake of brevity we report only the fall results here. This yielded two distinct factors, one composed of tests that loaded highly on reading-related predictor tests (namely, letter-sound and letter-name knowledge, blending and decoding in English) and one composed of tests with high loadings on language-related predictor tests (namely, receptive vocabulary, expressive morphology and sentence repetition in English). The emergence of these distinct factors is itself preliminary evidence that risk for reading and language difficulty constitute distinct profiles. We then standardized the scores on these tests and averaged the z-scores of the tests to

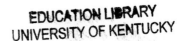

create two composite scores, one based on the reading predictor factor and one based on the language predictor factor. It was these composite average z-scores that were used in the discriminant analyses.

The reading composite predictor emerged as the more significant predictor of risk for pseudo-word decoding ability at the end of Grade 1 ($F(1,84) = 18.20$, $p < 0.001$), and was able to predict membership in the at-risk group with 88% accuracy and in the not-at-risk decoding group with 70% accuracy. The reading composite predictor was also a significant predictor of risk for reading comprehension ($F(1,84) = 22.35$, $p < 0.001$), and was able to predict membership in the at-risk group with 93% accuracy and in the not-at-risk group with 73% accuracy. The language composite predictor emerged as a significant predictor for language difficulty ($F(1,84) = 12.95$, $p < 0.001$). It was able to predict membership in the at-risk language subgroup with 69% accuracy and in the not-at-risk language subgroup with 82% accuracy.

In short, the results of these discriminant analyses reveal that risk for reading and language difficulties in an L2 are distinct profiles. At the same time, inspection of individual at-risk students revealed that, while most of them were at risk for reading difficulties only (41%) or language difficulties only (27%), some students were at risk for both reading and language difficulties (32%). These findings indicate that identification of L2 students who might be at risk for reading difficulty should include both reading- and language-related assessment in order to have comprehensive information about their strengths and weaknesses and, thus, of their intervention needs. Some students might require intervention that focuses only on reading, while other students may need intervention that includes language as well as reading support.

Taken together, the results of these analyses indicate that: (1) there is a core set of phonological processing weaknesses experienced by L2 readers who are at risk for word-decoding difficulties that have also been found in struggling L1 readers; (2) L2 reading comprehension difficulties appear to be associated with language-related deficits as well as word-decoding deficits, as has been found in L1 readers; (3) risk for L2 reading difficulties may be accompanied by risk for language difficulties, but the two are often distinct; and (4) it is possible to use L1 tests to predict risk for L2 reading and language difficulties, with moderate accuracy, up to almost two school years later.

Identification of Struggling L2 Readers

The identification of children with reading impairment, be they L1 or L2 students, is complex. This is due in part to the fact that multiple factors are associated with reading difficulty and these vary depending on whether the difficulty concerns word decoding or reading comprehension, as discussed earlier. An additional complexity in the case of L2 students is that it can be difficult to ascertain if a student's poor reading abilities are due to an under-lying impairment or inadequate opportunity or time to learn the language. This is particularly true for students who only begin to learn the L2 when they start school. As a result, educators often delay identification of reading impairment until students have had extended exposure to the L2 in order to rule out incomplete acquisition of the language as a contributing factor. However, a serious drawback to delaying identification, as noted earlier, is that critical intervention is also delayed.

An alternative approach to identifying L2 students with reading impair-ment that circumvents this problem is Response-to-Intervention (or RtI). RtI questions the need to distinguish an underlying impairment from other distal causes of reading difficulty, as proposed by the discrepancy approach, before intervention is implemented. In contrast, RtI recommends that addi-tional support be provided to all struggling readers, regardless of the cause of their difficulties. It also recommends that additional support be provided as soon as a student exhibits difficulties in learning to read relative to his/her peers. Early intervention makes it less likely that a student will develop sub-sequent ancillary problems that are linked to persistent reading difficulties, such as inability to keep up with academic instruction, low self-esteem and so on. Key to the RtI approach is the provision of successive 'tiers' of inter-vention for students who show persistent limited progress in response to intervention. Thus, progress monitoring is a key feature of this approach. Benchmark tests are often administered periodically following targeted intervention as formative assessments of students' response to intervention and of their ongoing needs (e.g. the Dynamic Indicators of Basic Early Literacy Skills (DIBELS) reading resources are frequently used for these pur-poses in the United States; https://dibels.uoregon.edu/). It is important when using benchmark or other standardized test instruments with L2 students that one does not use test norms based on the performance of native speakers uncritically, because they fail to reflect what is typical for L2 learners. If standardized or benchmark tests are used, the appropriate frame of reference for interpreting L2 students' results is the performance of other L2 students at the same stage of development and with the same exposure to the L2. Ultimately, approximation to native-speaker results is desirable, but it is inappropriate and invalid to use native-speaker norms as benchmarks for L2 students when they are just beginning the process of L2 acquisition.

The successive tiers of intervention that are provided for non-responsive students using an RtI approach become progressively more intense and indi-vidualized. To illustrate, in the case of students who begin school in K (around 5 years of age), the usual starting grade for children in North America, Tier 1 intervention is typically provided by classroom teachers in Grade 1 if a stu-dent has not shown adequate progress in response to classroom instruction in K. The results of our longitudinal study suggest that identification of at-risk L2 readers could begin as early as the fall of K even before students have had extensive L2 instruction, if assessment instruments that assess the core elements of reading are available in a student's L1. Tier 1 intervention usually involves high-quality, direct and individualized instruction by classroom teachers with a focus on the core elements of reading acquisition, including letter-sound knowledge, phonemic awareness, phonics and word decoding. The precise focus of instruction would depend on a student's specific needs. Subsequent benchmark testing after Tier 1 intervention would determine if a student continues to be non-responsive and thus qualifies for Tier 2 intervention. Evidence suggests that Tier 2 intervention should be provided in small classroom-based groups (Savage & Pompey, 2008) and should continue to include direct and systematic instruction of the core elements of reading, with plentiful opportunities to practice and receive feedback. It could also involve multi-sensory work with letters and sounds to strengthen the link between phonological and orthographic associations, which are often weak in at-risk readers (e.g. Hatcher, 2000; Hatcher *et al.*, 1994). Teaching to struggling readers' strengths is also recommended – for example, by focusing on their knowledge of vocabulary, morphology and semantics. Students who continue to be non-responsive after Tier 2 intervention, as determined by subsequent benchmark testing, would subsequently be provided with even more individualized, intensive intervention in one-on-one sessions in Tier 3 by remedial reading specialists.

Several arguments can be made in favor of an RtI approach. First, it avoids the problems associated with the wait-and-see strategy that is often associated with the traditional discrepancy model. Second, providing all struggling readers with early intervention is justifiable on the basis of research showing that there is a core set of cognitive, phonological and language-related abilities and processes that are associated with low reading performance regardless of the cause(s) of students' reading difficulties. Third, and in a related vein, these same findings would argue that all struggling readers would benefit from essentially the same core set of interventions, at least initially and taking individual differences into account. Finally, with specific reference to L2 readers who are at risk for reading impairment, by monitoring student progress over time in response to successive tiers of quality intervention that is tailored to their specific needs, an RtI approach makes it possible to rule out inadequate opportunity to acquire the L2 and/or inadequate prior reading instruction as a primary cause of L2 students' reading difficulties.

Notwithstanding the potential strengths and advantages of RtI, it is not without its problems and critics (e.g. Fuchs & Deshler, 2007; Savage & Deault, 2010). Critical to implementation of this approach is the identification of struggling readers who are not responsive to intervention. However, there is as yet no agreement, even in research on L1 reading development, as to what constitutes adequate growth in response to intervention (see Fuchs & Deshler, 2007, for a description of alternative methods of defining responsiveness in

English-L1 readers). Results from studies of Grade 1 English language learners in the United States suggest that monitoring change in L2 readers' oral reading fluency might be a useful way of gauging responsiveness to intervention (e.g. Al Otaiba *et al.*, 2009; Vaughn *et al.*, 2003). We are not aware of similar studies of response to intervention in higher grades. In the absence of definitive criteria for defining adequate response to intervention, each school or district may need to carry out its own action research to develop its own criteria or to critically examine those that have been proposed by others.

Additional concerns about RtI involve the nature and quality of effective intervention, both in Tier 1, which is widely assumed to include teacher-delivered instruction, and subsequently – in Tiers 2 and 3, when intervention is often provided by remediation specialists. With respect to Tier 1 intervention (or classroom instruction), Fuchs and Deschler (2007) point out that, while classroom teachers are encouraged to use 'scientifically validated' instruction to maximize reading development in all students, there is no empirical consensus concerning what this means. What constitutes effective intervention in Tiers 2 and 3 is equally unclear. Savage and Deault (2010) report that relatively short-term intervention focused on PA and phonics can be as effective as more extended intervention with struggling readers (Hatcher *et al.*, 2006; Torgesen, 2005). These findings call into question the value of extended interventions for struggling readers who are persistently non-responsive to intervention, as recommended by RtI. In addition, RtI often adopts a 'one-size-fits-all' approach and yet there is evidence that differentiated instruction is likely to be more effective with struggling readers (Juel & Minden-Cupp, 2000). How best to differentiate instruction is particularly important in the case of L2 students because, as noted earlier, these students often have varied cultural backgrounds, knowledge and expectations which, moreover, differ from those of mainstream students.

Conclusions

Assessment is crucial for identifying struggling L2 readers and for understanding their difficulties so that appropriate and effective intervention can be provided. Although we still have much to learn about L2 reading development, there is sufficient evidence at present, in our opinion, to guide educators' efforts to support struggling L2 readers. Evidence concerning the development of word decoding in L2 students, as in L1 students, is very robust and will undoubtedly grow. Current evidence strongly indicates a critical role for phonological processing (and PA in particular) and letter-sound knowledge in the development of word-decoding skills in both L1 and L2 reading development. Fortunately, there are readily available tests of these skills and knowledge that can be easily and efficiently administered by teachers and other education personnel; the tests and procedures we used in our own research are a good example. Research indicates further that indices of PA and letter-sound knowledge, along with RAN, can predict reading outcomes in either an L1 or an L2, both with respect to decoding and comprehension, up to two or even three years later. This evidence provides a solid basis for early identification of risk for L2 reading difficulties in the critical domain of decoding in either language.

Our own longitudinal research indicates that identification of risk for reading difficulty among L2 students can begin during the early stages of L2 acquisition, in K, using tests of these skills and knowledge in L2 students' native language, where such tests exist. When such tests are not available and thus tests that have been developed for native speakers of the L2 must be used, practitioners should avoid using native-speaker test norms for that language to interpret the results of L2 students. Expectations based on the performance of other similar L2 students are an appropriate point of comparison in these cases. While formal norms or standards for L2 students are not generally available, it is not unreasonable to imagine that school districts with large populations of L2 students might develop their own L2 norms. Briefly, this would entail testing a large number of L2 students with tests that provide relatively pure measures of word-decoding accuracy and fluency and reading comprehension in the L2. These results would then be used to determine the bottom 15th–20th percentile score, which could subsequently be used to identify struggling L2 readers who might qualify for additional support.

The evidence base for understanding the development of reading comprehension skills is much less complete than is the case for word decoding at this time. Nevertheless, it is clear that, along with word-decoding skills, knowledge of vocabulary, complex grammar and of text genre play critical roles in reading comprehension in both L1 and L2 students. Support for the significance of oral language in the development of reading comprehension skills comes from our own research findings (Erdos et al., 2011) that the SVR also applies to L2 reading comprehension. Although we still have much to learn about precisely what aspects of oral language competence influence the development of reading comprehension, and precisely how, there is sufficient evidence to recommend assessment of the oral language skills of L2 students who are struggling with reading comprehension. In contrast to the state of assessment of word-decoding ability and the components that underlie decoding ability, there is little agreement about what tests or measures are most suitable for the assessment of the oral language skills that support reading comprehension. In addition, critical analysis and use of reading comprehension tests is called for in order to identify and control the possible influence of confounding factors in reading tests, such as inordinate focus on word decoding, overemphasis on general knowledge, and cultural bias. In short, considerable judgment is called for in this respect.

RtI models offer a promising approach to the identification of (and planning interventions for) at-risk L2 readers. RtI appears to be particularly promising for these students, in our opinion, because it calls for early identification of and intervention for all students who are experiencing difficulty in learning to read, regardless of the source of their difficulty. This contrasts with the traditional discrepancy approach which often adopts a 'wait-and-see' strategy to ensure that students have an underlying reading impairment before individualized intervention is provided. RtI also has much to recommend for those working with L2 students because it includes an explicit strategy for fostering reading development over time, an important issue for many L2 students who need additional time to acquire the critical oral skills that underlie reading comprehension. Moreover, by including all struggling readers in early identification and intervention efforts, RtI is more equitable for L2 students who otherwise are often segregated from other students. Including classroom teachers in this process is also, we believe, desirable because it harnesses the talent and energy of everyone in the school who works with L2 students. Finally, because RtI recommends intervention and instruction that are informed by periodic and regular assessments of student progress, it advocates for a problem-solving curriculum-based approach to instruction, with assessment playing a critical and continuous role in all aspects of teaching and learning. These are all welcome innovations over traditional discrepancy or one-off clinical assessment models. RtI must, however, be understood and implemented critically. In particular, it should be implemented with a critical eye to the overall *quality* of the teaching and learning experiences of L2 students and not just phonics. Although much additional research is needed to fill gaps in our understanding of effective implementation of RtI, especially for L2 students, it has much to recommend for these students.

References

Al Otaiba, S., Petscher, Y., Pappamiheil, N.E., Williams, R.S., Dyrlund, A.K. and Connor, C. (2009) Modeling oral reading fluency development in Latino students: A longitudinal study across second and third grade. *Journal of Educational Psychology* 101 (3), 315–329.

August, D. and Hakuta, K. (1998) *Improving Schooling for Language Minority Children: A Research Agenda*. Washington, DC: National Academy Press.

August, D. and Shanahan, T. (2006) *Developing Literacy in Second Language Learners*. Report of the National Literacy Panel on Minority-Language Children and Youth. Mahwah, NJ: Lawrence Erlbaum.

Bialystok, E., Luk, G. and Kwan, E. (2005) Bilingualism, biliteracy, and learning to read: Interactions among languages and writing systems. *Scientific Studies of Reading* 9, 43–61.

Bishop, D.V.M. and Snowling, M.J. (2004) Developmental dyslexia and specific language: Same or different? *Psychological Bulletin* 130, 858–888.

Castles, A. and Nation, K. (2006) How does orthographic learning happen? In A. Castles and S. Andrews (eds) *From Inkmarks to Ideas: Challenges and Controversies About Word Recognition and Reading*. New York: Psychology Press.

Catts, H.W., Adlof, S.M., Hogan, T.P. and Weismer, S.E. (2005) Are specific language impairment and dyslexia distinct disorders? *Journal of Speech, Language and Hearing Research* 48, 1378–1396.

Catts, H.W., Gillespie, M., Leonard, L.B., Kail, R.V. and Miller, C.A. (2002) The role of speed of processing, rapid naming, and phonological awareness in reading achievement. *Journal of Learning Disabilities* 35, 509–524.

Chen, R. and Vellutino, F.R. (1997) Prediction of reading ability: A cross-validation study of the simple view of reading. *Journal of Literacy Research* 29 (1), 1–24.

Comaskey, E.M., Savage, R.S. and Abrami, P. (2009) A randomised efficacy study of web-based synthetic and analytic programmes among disadvantaged urban kindergarten children. *Journal of Research in Reading* 32 (1), 92–108.

Cormier, P., Desrochers, A. and Sénéchal, M. (2006) L'élaboration d'une batterie de tests en français pour l'évaluation des compétences en lecture. *Revue des Sciences de l'Éducation* 32, 205–225.

Deacon, S.H., Wade-Woolley, L. and Kirby, J. (2007) Crossover: The role of morphological awareness in French immersion children's reading. *Developmental Psychology* 43, 732–746.

DFES (2010a) English as an additional language: Introduction, accessed 2 April 2013. http://tesltoronto.org/international-students-in-canada-40-increase-since-2005

DFES (2010b) Key stage 2 results, accessed 2 April 2013. http://www.bdadyslexia.org.uk/about-dyslexia/further-information/dyslexia-research-information-.html

Dunn, L.M. and Dunn, L.M. (1997) *PPVT-III: Peabody Picture Vocabulary Test – Third Edition*. Circle Pines, MN: American Guidance Service.

Dunn, L.M., Thériault-Whalen, C.M. and Dunn, L.M. (1993) *Échelle de Vocabulaire en Images Peabody – EVIP*. Toronto: Psycan.

Erdos, C., Genesee, F., Savage, R. and Haigh, C. (2011) Individual differences in second language reading outcomes. *International Journal of Bilingualism* 15 (1), 3–25.

Erdos, C., Genesee, F., Savage, R. and Haigh, C. (in press) Predicting risk for oral and written language learning difficulties in students educated in a second language. *Applied Psycholinguistics*. doi: 10.1017/S0142716412000422.

Fuchs, D. and Deshler, D.D. (2007) What we need to know about responsiveness to intervention (and shouldn't be afraid to ask). *Learning Disabilities Research and Practice* 22, 129–136.

Garnett, B. (2006) An introductory look at the academic trajectories of ESL students. Paper presented at the Immigration, Integration and Language Conference, 11 October 2006, University of Calgary.

Genesee, F. (2007) French immersion and at-risk students: A review of research findings. *Canadian Modern Language Review* 63, 655–688.

Genesee, F. and Geva, E. (2006) Cross-linguistic relationships in working memory, phonological processes, and oral language. In D. August and T. Shanahan (eds) *Developing Literacy in Second Language Learners. Report of the National Literacy Panel on Minority-Language Children and Youth* (pp. 175–184). Mahwah, NJ: Lawrence Erlbaum.

Genesee, F. and Jared, D. (2008) Literacy development in early French immersion programs. *Canadian Psychology* 49, 140–147.

Genesee, F. and Lindholm-Leary, K. (2012) The education of English language learners. In K. Harris, S. Graham and T. Urdan *et al.* (eds) *APA Handbook of Educational Psychology* (pp. 499–526). Washington, DC: APA Books.

Genesee, F., Lindholm-Leary, K., Saunders, W. and Christian, D. (2006) *Educating English Language Learners: A Synthesis of Research Evidence*. New York: Cambridge University Press.

Gersten, R. and Geva, E. (2003) Teaching reading to early language learners. *Educational Leadership* 60 (7), 44–49.

Geva, E. and Clifton, S. (1994) The development of first and second language reading skills in early French immersion. *Canadian Modern Language Review* 50, 646–667.

Gonzalez, N., Moll, L.C. and Amanti, C. (2005) *Funds of Knowledge: Theorizing Practices in Household, Communities and Classrooms.* Mahwah, NJ: Lawrence Erlbaum.

Gough, P.B. and Tunmer, W.E. (1986) Decoding, reading and reading disability. *Remedial and Special Education 77,* 6–10.

Gutiérrez-Clellen, V.F., Simon-Cereijido, G. and Wagner, C. (2008) Bilingual children with language impairment: A comparison with monolinguals and second language learners. *Applied Psycholinguistics 29,* 3–19.

Haigh, C., Savage, R.S., Erdos, C. and Genesee, F. (2011) The role of phoneme and onset-rime awareness in second language reading acquisition. *Journal of Research in Reading* (Special issue: Learning to read in more than one language) 34 (1), 94–113.

Hatcher, P. (2000) Sound links in reading and spelling with discrepancy-defined dyslexics and children with moderate learning difficulties. *Reading and Writing* 13, 257–272.

Hatcher, P.J., Hulme, C. and Ellis, A.W. (1994) Ameliorating early reading failure by integrating the teaching of reading and phonological skills: The phonological linkage hypothesis. *Child Development* 65, 41–57.

Hatcher, P.J., Hulme, C., Miles, J.N., Carroll, J.M., Hatcher, J., Gibbs, S., *et al.* (2006) Efficacy of small group reading intervention for beginning readers with reading-delay: A randomized control trial. *Journal of Child Psychology and Psychiatry* 47, 820–827.

Hoover, W.A. and Gough, P.B. (1990) The simple view of reading. *Reading and Writing: An Interdisciplinary Journal* 2, 127–160.

Jared, D., Cormier, P., Levy, B.A. and Wade-Woolley, L. (2011) Early predictors of biliteracy development in children in French immersion: A 4-year longitudinal study. *Journal of Educational Psychology* 103 (1), 119–139.

Joshi, R.M. and Aaron, P.G. (2000) The component model of reading: Simple view of reading made a little more complex. *Reading Psychology* 21, 85–97.

Juel, C. and Minden-Cupp, C. (2000) Learning to read words: Linguistic units and instructional strategies. *Reading Research Quarterly* 35 (4), 458–488.

Keenan, J.M. and Betjemann, R.S. (2006) Comprehending the Gray Oral Reading Test without reading it: Why comprehension tests should not include passage-independent items. *Scientific Studies of Reading* 10, 363–380.

Kirby, J.R. and Savage, R.S. (2008) Can the simple view deal with the complexities of reading? *Literacy* 42, 75–82.

Lesaux, N., Crosson, A.C., Kieffer, M.J. and Pierce, M. (2010) Uneven profiles: Language minority learners' word reading, vocabulary, and reading comprehension skills. *Journal of Applied Developmental Psychology* 31, 475–483.

Lesaux, N. and Geva, E. with Koda, K., Siegel, L. and Shanahan, T. (2008) Development of literacy in second-language learners. In D. August and T. Shanhan (eds) *Developing Reading and Writing in Second Language Learners* (pp. 27–60). New York: Routledge, Center for Applied Linguistics and International Reading Association.

Lesaux, N.K. and Kieffer, M. (2010) Exploring sources of reading comprehension difficulties among language minority learners and their classmates in early adolescence. *American Educational Research Journal* 47 (3), 596–632.

Lesaux, N.K. and Siegel, L.S. (2003) The development of reading in children who speak English as a second language. *Developmental Psychology* 3 (6), 1005–1019.

Mathes, P.G., Pollard-Durodola, S.D., Cardenas-Hagan, E., Linan-Thompson, S. and Vaughn, S. (2007) Teaching struggling readers who are native Spanish speakers: What do we know? *Language, Speech and Hearing Services in Schools* 38, 260–271.

Muter, V., Hulme, C., Snowling, M.J. and Stevenson, J. (2004) Phonemes, rimes and language skills as foundations of early reading development: Evidence from a longitudinal study. *Developmental Psychology* 40, 663–681.

Nation, K. (2005) Children's reading comprehension difficulties. In M.J. Snowling and C. Hulme (eds) *The Science of Reading: A Handbook* (pp. 248–265). Oxford: Blackwell.

Nation, K. and Snowling, M. (1997) Assessing reading difficulties: The validity and utility of current measures of reading skill. *British Journal of Educational Psychology* 67, 359–370.

National Center for Education Statistics (2007) *The Condition of Education 2007* (NCES 2007-064). Washington, DC: US Government Printing Office. http://nces.ed.gov/pubs2007/2007064.pdf.

NICHD (2002) National Institute of Child Health & Human Development website. http://www.nichd.nih.gov/.

Oakhill, J., Cain, K. and Bryant, P.E. (2003) The dissociation of word reading and text comprehension: Evidence from component skills. *Language and Cognitive Processes* 18, 443–468.

Obadia, A. and Thériault, C.M.L. (1997) Attrition in French immersion programs: Possible solutions. *Canadian Modern Language Review* 53, 506–529.

OECD (2006) *Where Immigrant Students Succeed – A Comparative Review of Performance and Engagement in PISA 2003*. OECD Publishing. http://www.oecd.org.

Paradis, J., Crago, M., Genesee, F. and Rice, M. (2003) Bilingual children with specific language impairment: How do they compare with their monolingual peers? *Journal of Speech, Language and Hearing Research* 46, 1–15 (Figure erratum).

Paradis, J., Genesee, F. and Crago, M.B. (2011) *Dual Language Development and Disorders: A Handbook on Bilingualism and Second Language Learning* (2nd edn). Baltimore, MD: Brookes Publishing.

Perfetti, C. (2003) The universal grammar of reading. *Scientific Studies of Reading* 7, 3–24.

Perfetti, C. (2007) Reading ability: Lexical quality to comprehension. *Scientific Studies of Reading* 11, 357–384.

Rice, L. and Wexler, K. (2001) *Test for Early Grammatical Impairment: Examiner's Manual*. San Antonio, TX: Psychological Corporation/Harcourt Assessment.

Riches, C. and Genesee, F. (2006) Cross-linguistic and cross-modal aspects of literacy development. In F. Genesee, K. Lindholm-Leary, W. Saunders and D. Christian (eds) *Educating English Language Learners: A Synthesis of Research Evidence* (pp. 64–108). New York: Cambridge University Press.

Sanchez, K.S., Bledsoe, L.M., Sumabat, C. and Ye, R. (2004) Hispanic students' reading situations and problems. *Journal of Hispanic Higher Education* 3 (1), 50–63.

Savage, R. (2006) Effective early reading instruction and inclusion: Some reflections on mutual dependence. *International Journal of Inclusive Education: Special Issue* 10, 347–361.

Savage, R.S., Carless, S. and Ferrero, V. (2007) Predicting curriculum and test performance from pupil background, baseline skills and phonological awareness at age 5: A six-year follow-up at the end of Key Stage 2. *Journal of Child Psychology and Psychiatry* 48 (7), 732–739.

Savage, R.S. and Deault, L. (2010) Understanding and supporting children experiencing dyslexia and ADHD: The challenge of constructing models incorporating constitutional and classroom influences. In K. Littleton, C. Wood and J.K. Staarman, (eds) *International Handbook of Psychology in Education* (pp. 569–608). Bingley: Emerald.

Savage, R.S. and Pompey, Y. (2008) What does the evidence really say about effective literacy teaching? *Educational and Child Psychology* 25 (3), 17–26.

Savage, R. and Wolforth, J. (2007) An additive simple view of reading describes the performance of good and poor readers in higher education. *Exceptionality Education Canada* 17 (2), 243–268.

Scanlon, D.M., Anderson, K.L. and Flynn, L.H. (2008a) *Preventing Reading Difficulties: The Role of Instruction and Experience Before First Grade*. Presentation for the Early Childhood Direction Center, Capital Region Board of Cooperative Educational Services, Latham, NY.

Scanlon, D.M., Gelzheiser, L.M., Vellutino, F.R., Schatschneider, C. and Sweeney, J.M. (2008b) Reducing the incidence of early reading difficulties: Professional development for classroom teachers vs. direct interventions for children. *Learning and Individual Differences* 18, 346–359.

Semel, E.M., Wiig, E.H. and Secord, W. (2003) *Clinical Evaluation of Language Fundamentals* (CELF-4). San Antonio, TX: Psychological Corporation.

Share, D.L. (2008) Orthographic learning, phonology and the self-teaching hypothesis. In R. Kail (ed.) *Advances in Child Development and Behavior.* San Diego, CA: Elsevier Academic Press.

Shatil, E. and Share, D.L. (2003) Cognitive antecedents of early reading ability: A test of the modularity hypothesis. *Journal of Experimental Child Psychology* 86 (1), 1–31.

Shaywitz, S.E. and Shaywitz, B.A. (2005) Neurobiological indices of dyslexia. In H.L. Swanson, K.R. Harris and S. Graham (eds) *Handbook of Learning Disabilities* (pp. 514–531). New York: Guilford Press.

Snowling, M.J. (2000) *Dyslexia.* Oxford: Blackwell.

Statistics Canada (2004) Literacy scores, human capital and growth across fourteen OECD countries. Monograph No. 11, 89–552-MIE. Ottawa: Statistics Canada, accessed 2 April 2013. http://www.dyslexiaassociation.ca/english/about.shtml

Torgesen, J.K. (2005) Remedial interventions for students with dyslexia: National goals and current accomplishments. In Richardson, S. and Gilger, J. (eds) *Research-Based Education and Intervention: What We Need to Know* (pp. 103–124). Boston, MA: International Dyslexia Association.

Vaughn, S., Linan-Thompson, S. and Hickman-Davis, P. (2003) Response to instruction as a means of identifying students with reading/learning disabilities. *Exceptional Children* 69, 391–410.

Vaughn, S., Linan-Thompson, S., Pollard-Durodola, S.D., Mathes, P.G. and Cardenas-Hagan, E. (2006) Effective intervention for English language learners (Spanish–English) at risk for reading difficulties. In D.K. Dickinson and S.B. Neuman (eds) *Handbook of Early Literacy Research* (Vol. 2; pp. 185–197). New York: Guildford Press.

Wallach, G.P. (2007) *Language Intervention for School-age Students: Setting Goals for Academic Success.* St. Louis, MI: Mosby Elsevier.

Wechsler, D. (2005) *Wechsler Individual Achievement Test 2nd Edition* (WIAT II). London: Psychological Corporation.

Wilkinson, G.S. (1993) *The Wide Range Achievement Test: Manual* (3rd edn). Wilmington, DE: Wide Range.

Willms, D. and Murray, S. (2007) *International Adult Literacy Survey: Gaining and Losing Literacy Skills Over the Lifecourse.* Ottawa: Statistics Canada.

Ziegler, J.C. and Goswami, U.C. (2005) Reading acquisition, developmental dyslexia, and skilled reading across languages: A Psycholinguistic Grain Size theory. *Psychological Bulletin* 131, 3–29.

3 What Are the Building Blocks for Language Acquisition? Underlying Principles of Assessment for Language Impairment in the Bilingual Context

Carolyn Letts

This chapter considers the assessment of the acquisition of spoken language in young bilingual children within the context of potential language impairment. The main focus is on the use of assessment to identify language impairment, and in particular the use of formal test procedures. The difficulties surrounding such assessment are explored. This is followed by a discussion of the extent to which it is possible to develop assessments that reflect stages and skills that are of significance in the acquisition of any language. Linguistic features that have been associated with language impairment are also discussed, again against the backdrop of potential universality. Finally, suggestions are made regarding the development of assessment procedures for early language abilities in children acquiring language in a bi- or multilingual context.

Introduction

An important context in which it may be necessary to assess the language ability of a bilingual child is that of speech and language therapy (SLT, sometimes referred to as speech language pathology). In this context oral language ability is the main focus of attention, although written language may be of interest where older children are concerned. One of the main requirements of such assessment is the identification of a potential underlying difficulty with language acquisition, that is to say, the presence of an overall language delay or impairment. Such a difficulty will have an impact on the child's acquisition of all the languages to which he or she is exposed and will not be limited to second language learning. Although conditions such as deafness, neurological damage or disorder, severe environmental deprivation, generalized learning disability and autistic spectrum disorder are known to impair language acquisition, in many cases in which the child is slow to acquire language skills the cause is unknown. This is captured in the defining features of *specific language impairment* (SLI) or *primary language impairment*, where the possible etiological factors listed above are all excluded from the child's diagnostic profile (Leonard, 1998). Identification in these instances depends on establishing that the child's language development is significantly behind, or significantly different from, that of age peers who share the same linguistic background. This chapter will focus on assessment for this purpose, concentrating on oral language abilities in young children (toddlers to early school years). In particular, issues concerning the adaptation of standardized and/or formal test procedures for use with children in bilingual contexts will be addressed. As there is considerable overlap between the linguistic characteristics of SLI and those of other language impairments that do not reach strict exclusion criteria (that is, there may be additional non-linguistic impairments involved), the preferred term for this sort of communication difficulty as used here will be *language impairment* (LI).

While the mere fact of being bilingual does not in itself impact negatively on language acquisition, bilingual children are as much at risk for LI as the monolingual population. The report produced by Bercow (2008), drawing on work published by Lindsay *et al.* in 2010, estimates that 7% of children in the UK have speech, language and communication needs (SLCN). In situations where significant proportions of children are living in bi- or multilingual communities, some children with SLCN will therefore inevitably be bilingual.

Professionals such as speech and language therapists (SLTs) have a number of specific aims they need to fulfil when assessing children. Crucially, they have to identify children who are at risk for communication impairment. This is done by comparing their communicative behaviour, including language comprehension and production, with that of their age peers: where they appear to be lagging behind significantly, this may indicate a problem requiring help and intervention if the child's educational, social and personal development is to remain uncompromised. Once an impairment is identified, further assessment is required to build up a profile of language ability, to identify aspects and areas that have the greatest developmental impact on the child, and to plan intervention and to measure progress (Cupples, 2011).

In the bilingual context, SLTs are faced with a number of issues that do not apply when working with monolingual children. Some of these are:

(1) *Diversity within bilingual populations.* The ways in which children become bilingual and the degree of exposure they have had to each language vary enormously. The expectations regarding acquisition of each language for a child who has been exposed to two languages from birth, for example, will be very different from what might be expected if the child has only recently been exposed to a second language. When one language is clearly a second language (L2) for the child, the length of exposure and contexts in which s/he uses the language will have to be taken into account. This means that identifying an appropriate peer group for comparison is important, but can be difficult.

(2) *Lack of norms.* The majority of normative information on language acquisition relates to English. Where information is available for other languages, this is most frequently within the context of monolingualism. Information is beginning to emerge regarding bilingual language acquisition, suggesting that there may be lags in comparison to monolingual acquisition in some areas (vocabulary, morphosyntax) when each language is viewed in isolation, with catch-up at a later point (see, for example, Gathercole & Thomas, 2009; Hoff *et al.*, 2012; Paradis, 2010). This suggests that direct comparison with monolingual norms is not advisable.

(3) *Lack of knowledge.* Professionals are often not bilingual themselves and will in most instances not be speakers of one or more of the child's languages. It may be difficult to get information about characteristics of a child's home language(s), for example, if the variety spoken is low status and/or has no written form (see Pert & Letts, 2006, for an example of this). In addition, code-switching may be commonplace in the child's community, or may be a rare feature in a home where parents try to keep each language separate. Information will therefore be needed on whether code-switching should occur and what form this may take. This will help a professional assess whether switches on the child's part are a common element of that child's experience with the two languages or fall outside that experience, and therefore whether the child can be expected to display code-switching in their expressive language.

(4) *Risk of confusion with characteristics of second language acquisition (SLA).* Practitioners will often be familiar with one of the languages that the child is acquiring (for example in the UK, English, if this is a language the child is acquiring in school). This will, however, often be a non-dominant second language for the child, who will understandably be behind his monolingual English-speaking age peers. Especially with very young children whose knowledge of one of their languages may be limited, it is always advisable to assess in all the languages to which the

child is exposed. De Jong and colleagues have done extensive work to disentangle features associated with SLA from those associated with SLI in children who are bilingual Turkish–Dutch speakers. However, they have found many areas of overlap between the two groups when looking at children's second language (de Jong *et al.*, 2010; Orgassa, 2009).

In addition to all of the above issues, cultural differences between the professional and the child's family may impose further barriers and increase the potential for misunderstandings and misinterpretation of assessment outcomes (see Isaac, 2002, for further information in this area).

The aim of this chapter is to take the reader through aspects and stages of language acquisition that should be worthy of assessment regardless of the linguistic background of the child, while keeping in mind all these issues. Strategies are offered that will aid in devising assessment procedures and materials.

Assessment Techniques

A number of different tools and techniques are used by SLTs for assessment, including observation, language sampling, informal probes and formal tests. The techniques of choice will vary according to the stage in the assessment and intervention cycle; specific criterion-referenced probes, for example, may be most useful after a period of intervention, in order to evaluate what the child has learned and how effective the intervention has been. When at the earlier stage of identifying the child who may be at risk, a range of tools are ideally used to build up a comprehensive picture (Cupples, 2011). Observation of children in different social settings will give a picture of their interaction with age peers and with adults, and of the impact of any communication impairment on educational and social activities. This initial impression will then be explored more thoroughly, often with formal testing. The formal test offers a structured framework that can be worked through systematically. At this stage, tests that sample a range of key language behaviours are useful, as too specific a focus on one level of language (e.g. vocabulary or morphology) may result in the missing of difficulties at other levels. Formal published tests may be available (in which case the materials will look professional and be durable) and, importantly, they will often be standardized on a normative sample. This provides ready comparison with age peers. Testers are encouraged to check standardized tests for a number of features before using them – for example, the representativeness of the normative sample; reliability and validity; and ability to discriminate between children who have language difficulty and those who do not (sensitivity and specificity). Lidz (2003) describes these features of standardized tests in the context of children with special educational needs, as well as discussing other types of assessment procedure. (See also Chapter 6 by Peña *et al.*, this volume.)

While formal and standardized tests have a number of advantages, especially in terms of controlling the linguistic features that are sampled, they also have a number of inherent drawbacks. Children may be unfamiliar with the 'test' situation and unnerved by it and so may not perform well. Furthermore, tests are good for illustrating what children appear unable to do, but they do not address *why* they have failed certain items (i.e. is it because of genuine lack of language competence or the result of being bored or distracted?), nor do they reveal what children *can* do. For these reasons, it is recommended that test results be complemented both by language sampling and by further investigation of areas of language that seem problematic.

Testing Bilingual Children

Important features of tests: Standardization and theoretical basis

There are very few standardized tests that have been developed for children who are bilingual. Such development involves norming on a sufficiently large sample of typically developing bilingual children, who are grouped according to similar linguistic and social backgrounds. Large numbers may be difficult to locate and, because of the diversity of background mentioned above, the norming sample may differ in important ways from any individual child who is subsequently tested. Tests that have been developed in such a way include *Prawf Geirfa Cymraeg* (Welsh–English vocabulary; see Gathercole *et al.*, 2008), *Sandwell Bilingual Screening Assessment Scales for Expressive Punjabi and English* (Duncan *et al.*, 1988), and the *Test of Auditory Comprehension of Language. English/Spanish* (Carrow, 1973).

While standardization is the most obvious and most often mentioned problem around creating tests for the bilingual child population, a further issue relates to the theoretical premises on which the test is developed. The minimal requirement is that the test reflect important linguistic features that are associated with the target age group; for tests that cover a wide age range and a number of developmental stages, this will include a number of such features. Selection of these features will depend very much on the state of knowledge, both theoretical and empirical, at the time the test is developed. The *Reynell Developmental Language Scales* (RDLS), for example, which are used extensively in the UK, were developed in the 1960s and have since undergone a number of transformations with each new edition. Throughout, the target age group has been the preschool and early primary school population (between 18 months and 7 years 6 months, although there have been minor changes to the exact age range over time). Early editions were based on experience arising from clinical practice, and they featured aspects of language that appeared to be important both for typical language acquisition and for impaired children who had language delays or disorders. Reynell (1977) incorporated a large normative sample of typically developing children, so that it was then possible to make confident predictions about normal stages of language acquisition *in English*; there was no consideration of developmental profiles in other languages, and the standardization sample consisted of children who were all monolingual English speakers.

Subsequent editions of RDLS (*RDLS-III*; Edwards *et al.*, 1997, and the *New RDLS* (*NRDLS*; Edwards *et al.*, 2011) incorporated advances in knowledge in two areas, first, relative to stages of language acquisition, and second, with regard to key features of LI. These advances were fuelled, first, by the blossoming of research on child language acquisition from the 1970s onwards and the development of tools such as *LARSP* (*Linguistic Assessment, Remediation and Screening Procedure*; Crystal *et al.*, 1976), which enabled comparison of a young child's language acquisition with specific age-related stages. The second major influence, more apparent in *NRDLS* (2011), was the search for linguistic 'markers' of child LI, and especially *specific* language impairment (SLI: see above). The earliest research in this area was conducted in the area of the acquisition of morphology, especially verb morphology, following seminal work by Rice and colleagues (Rice, 2003). Subsequent areas that have been considered have been complex sentences, object clitics, and pronouns (e.g. Van der Lely & Stollwerck, 1997), as well as processing skills reflected in non-word repetition (e.g. Archibald & Gathercole, 2006; Chiat & Roy, 2007) and sentence repetition tasks (e.g. Riches *et al.*, 2010).

While it can be argued that the theoretical rationale behind some formal test procedures is becoming increasingly sophisticated, there has been little consideration until comparatively recently of the universality of such rationales across different linguistic contexts. Indeed, there is a 'tradition' within test development to exclude children who are bilingual from any normative sample, because they will necessarily be different and, therefore, risk skewing results. Importantly, though, those aspects of language known to be difficult for LI children have increasingly been the subject of crosslinguistic studies of children with SLI, and so we have some information on the degree to which the difficulties are language-specific or might be common to SLI children from a range of language backgrounds. For example, studies have been conducted looking at verb morphology (e.g. Bortolini *et al.*, 2002; Dromi *et al.*, 1999; Hansson & Leonard, 2003; Roberts & Leonard, 1997), pronouns (e.g. Stavrakaki & Van der Lely, 2010), complex sentences (e.g. Novadgradsky & Friedmann, 2006), and passives (e.g. Leonard *et al.*, 2006).

Basis for bilingual assessment: Stages of language acquisition

As indicated in the previous section, a good formal assessment procedure will include tasks and sections that reflect key stages in the language acquisition process and/or items that are known to be problematic for children with LI. While studies of language acquisition in a range of languages have been increasing, it is still the case that the overwhelming majority of work done in this area, and certainly the focus of the main textbooks (e.g. Berko-Gleason & Ratner, 2009; Hoff, 2005; Hulit & Howard, 2005), is based on acquisition of English. An important question then is to what extent these stages of language acquisition are 'universal', applying both to languages other than English in the monolingual context, and to bilingual acquisition. For individual languages and language combinations this question can be addressed by extensive data collection from young typically developing children, but this research takes considerable time; clinicians and other professionals working to identify LI children require something that is available currently on which to base their judgments. A common strategy is to translate (or better, adapt) a test or procedure that is already available, usually in English, while recognizing that the information gleaned in this way should be treated with caution because of issues related to the very different populations on which the test was standardized. This still leaves the problem of how universal the stages of language acquisition represented by the test might be.

Letts and Sinka (2011) have produced a *Multilingual Toolkit* to accompany *NRDLS*. This gives guidelines for those who are contemplating trying to adapt the test for use in languages other than English, and for use in bilingual contexts. In preparing this, an attempt has been made to indicate features of language acquisition that are arguably universal, and also features that are hard to learn and therefore potentially at risk when the child is language impaired. The following assumptions are made about universal sequences of language acquisition:

(1) Comprehension and production of single words come before comprehension and production of multi-word utterances. Children who are late to acquire single words are at risk for LI.
(2) Early sentences are simple and consist of verbs with accompanying argument structures. Where children are slow to move on to multi-word utterances and produce simple sentences, they are likely to be at risk for LI.
(3) Comprehension and production of sentences that are complex in various ways (e.g. contain embedded clauses, or feature 'movement') develop later than comprehension and production of simple sentences. Older children who have LI are likely to have more difficulty with complex sentences, when compared to age peers.
(4) The integrated skills required for inferential understanding and for making metalinguistic judgements are relatively late to develop. In children with LI, these skills will be particularly slow. While there is some evidence for different processing systems in bilingual children leading

at times to an advantage in metalinguistic tasks (see, for example, Bialystok, 1991), there have been no studies that indicate a corresponding mitigation of delay in the development of metalinguistic skills in bilingual children who have LI.

A comprehensive assessment of language acquisition would be expected to reflect these assumptions. Other aspects of acquisition that are undoubtedly important in many languages may not be universal in the same way. Verb morphology, for example, is present with varying degrees of richness in many languages in Europe, for example, but may be absent or all but absent elsewhere, such as in the languages of China. Locative marking, generally expressed through prepositional phrases in English, is known to be expressed by a variety of other linguistic devices in other languages; Dabrowska (2004) lists adpositions, nouns, adverbs, particles, verbs, adjectives, verb affixes and noun inflections as all potentially fulfilling this function. This means that linguistic complexity for expressing location will vary across languages, and children learning distinct languages may be at different ages/stages before they can understand and talk about location correctly.

The stages embodied in the assumptions listed above feel intuitively obvious, in that there is a development from comparatively simple structures (single words) to more complex ones (e.g. complex sentences). Further empirical support for this progression was provided during the trialling stage of *NRDLS.* A large number of test items, divided into appropriate sections, were trialled on a sample of 301 children in the age range of 18 months to 7 years 6 months. In order to maximize the number of items that could be trialled without exhausting the patience of the participants, children were divided into two groups, each of which took different versions of the test. Each section had a number of anchor items, common to both versions, plus items that were unique to the particular version. The anchor items served as common points to which the relative difficulty of non-anchor items could be compared. Sections and items could then be evaluated on a number of factors including internal reliability, ability to discriminate between children of different ages, and progressive development with age across the test. It was then possible to construct a test consisting of coherent sections ordered according to difficulty. The youngest children were quite successful in completing the sections involving selecting or naming objects (nouns) but were unable to score on other sections. The most difficult sections were those involving inferential meaning and grammaticality judgment (involving metalinguistic awareness), for which only the oldest children in the sample (around ages 5 years 6 months to 7 years) were successful. The resulting ordering of sections reflected the broad ordering suggested above, *for English.* Moreover, for English, sections are included that cover English verb morphology and prepositions expressing spatial relationships. For different languages and in the bilingual context, different ordering may be expected in terms of where such sections would be placed, or indeed whole sections may be irrelevant. Even within the broadest stages listed above, there may also be variation in acquisition across languages. Early single word vocabulary for children speaking some languages may contain a relatively high proportion of verbs in comparison to English and other languages where there is an early 'noun bias' (see, for example, Choi & Gopnik, 1995; Kim et al., 2000). This may affect the way early vocabulary is assessed for these languages.

When considering children who are developing language in a bilingual context, these broad stages would still be expected to apply; however, the possibility of a lag in development in any one language then needs to be considered. With vocabulary, for example, bilingual children may have a lower vocabulary than monolingual age peers for each language, but their total vocabulary or total conceptual vocabulary needs to be considered (Patterson, 1998; Peña et al., 2002), as well as potential cognate or borrowed items across the two languages (Chapter 7 by Stadthagen-González et al., this volume). A further consideration is intra-sentential code switching which may occur (Pert & Letts, 2006; Paradis et al., 2000) in multiword utterances. Any assessment would need to allow for this and for mixed or code-switched utterances to be credited accordingly.

Basis for bilingual assessment: Indicators of language impairment

Besides drawing on developmental stages in acquisition, the other area that may drive language assessment is that of potential markers of LI. As indicated above, crosslinguistic studies have searched for these, for example, in the areas of verb morphology and complex sentences. English-speaking children with SLI are known to find tense marking difficult, specifically third person singular (present tense) -s and past tense -ed. Studies looking at how SLI children cope with verb inflections in different languages have indicated variation in the degree of difficulty with tense and person markers, which can often be plausibly explained by characteristics of the target language (see, for example, Bedore & Leonard, 2005; Kunnari et al., 2011; Thordardottir, 2008). Where verb morphology is comparatively rich (i.e. all verb forms are inflected in some way, so the child does not have to remember which ones are affected) and also regular, children acquire the morphology earlier and these inflections are less problematic for children with SLI. The field cannot yet identify exactly which types of structures, under which circumstances, are particularly difficult for children with LI. Among the clear indicators of a problem that is unlikely to resolve are the severity of a delay and the presence of difficulty in comprehending language as well as producing it. Beyond this, however, with current knowledge, it would be wise to incorporate some of the aspects thought to be vulnerable into any assessment. There is evidence that intervention can be effective with young children (see review by Cable & Domsch, 2011), and also that LIs can have long-lasting damaging effects on the child's later educational and social development. The arguments for identifying the problem and intervening as early as possible are therefore persuasive, although it has also been noted that a significant number of preschool children with expressive language delays may improve spontaneously (Law *et al.*, 2000).

It is important to bear in mind, however, that, while areas identified as potential markers of LI appear to be powerful indicators of LI, they also tend to be more complex, and therefore later developing, aspects of language structure. As part of the process of standardizing *NRDLS*, for example, a group of 35 LI children, as diagnosed by SLTs, aged between 4 years 6 months and 7 years 6 months, were compared with children matched for gender and age from the main normative sample. Significant differences in scores were found for both comprehension and production. LI children had particular difficulty with producing complex sentences. However, this was a section that even typically developing children found difficult – they were found to be able to perform competently only when they were around 5 years 6 months. (Note that they can produce some of these structures spontaneously before that age.) It is clear, then, that the use of complex sentences would not work as an indicator of impairment in younger children. Assessments that tap into earlier stages, including single word vocabulary, early two-word utterances and simple sentences are therefore required.

Adapting Tests

The following sections concern the development and/or adaptation of formal tests in line with different linguistic contexts, focusing on single words, simple sentences and complex sentences. It is assumed that these aspects of language acquisition would form the basic substance of a test that, like *NRDLS*, samples a variety of language behaviours and is developmental – that is to say, accommodates a range of ages. There are also procedures that focus on particular aspects of language (e.g. vocabulary or syntax), or particular age ranges, or both. These will be mentioned where relevant. For guidelines for adapting *NRDLS* specifically to non-English contexts, please refer to Letts and Sinka (2011).

In many ways, the ideal approach for developing tests in other languages is to use research evidence to develop items tailored for each language situation, without reference to test materials available for other languages. Evidence from the wider research literature on testing can be used to inform the framework for test construction (as is suggested above with reference to possible universal stages of development), but individual items can be constructed in line with the cultural and environmental experience of the target population and the linguistic characteristics of the target language(s). However, in clinical and educational situations, professionals often do not have that luxury and need something that can be used immediately. So there may be a need to adapt materials and resources to which the assessing professional already has access. The following sections will aim to give suggestions for both these scenarios.

Early single words

The understanding and production of single words are the very earliest language skills that can be demonstrated through a formal procedure, usually through asking the child to choose a picture or object from a wider selection according to a word s/he hears (comprehension) or to name a picture or object. Care must be taken that the vocabulary sampled is likely to be within the young child's experience and that there is evidence that young children know these words and regularly use them. Where existing materials are adapted, translation equivalents may be problematic. There may be more than one lexical item available, so a choice must be made. For example, Latvian has a direct equivalent of the English word *pencil*, but a generic term *rakstāmais* (meaning 'writing instrument') is also widely used. Alternatively, a single lexical item may not exist that exactly captures the meaning of the item; for example, with Welsh-speaking children a phrase *codi llaw*, literally 'lift hand', is commonly used where English speakers would use the verb *wave*.

If the focus of assessment is exclusively on early vocabulary, there may be other resources that might give a clearer picture of the child's capacity in this area. A naturalistic language sample could yield a type-token ratio or 'D' measure of vocabulary diversity (Malvern & Richards, 2002). This gives an indication of the range of vocabulary used by the child in spontaneous language and of the degree to which the child can exploit different vocabulary items in the structures he or she produces. The McArthur–Bates Communicative Development Inventories (CDI) checklists completed by parents about their child's early language, especially early words, have been developed for a broad range of languages and linguistic contexts. An example developed in the bilingual context of Malta is that of Gatt (Gatt *et al.*, 2008; see also Chapter 4 by Ezeizabarrena *et al.*, this volume; Chapter 5 by O'Toole, this volume). For further examples, see the McArthur–Bates CDI website (http://www.sci.sdsu.edu/cdi/adaptations_ol.htm). Both language sampling and use of checklists have the advantage that bilingual situations can be easily accommodated. Since they tap into naturalistic use, whichever language is appropriate to the situation can be used, including code-switching and code-switched varieties. Alternatively, these resources may be used as sources for identifying suitable lexical items for an early vocabulary section on a broader test. Naturalistic language samples for a range of language situations can be found on the CHILDES website (http://childes.psy.cmu.edu/).

A further consideration arises if one wishes to tap into word classes beyond nouns. Noun vocabulary is relatively easy to elicit or test for comprehension in the formal test situation, as concrete objects or pictures can be used. Verb vocabulary is rather more difficult, but it is possible to develop sections on verbs, as for *NRDLS*, by animating toys and by using pictures of activities. While other word classes do of course feature in the early vocabularies of children, there is evidence that, in many languages, nouns make up a large proportion of early words (the so-called 'noun-bias') and so sampling nouns should give an insight into the child's progress. The test developer needs to be sensitive, however, to the evidence (cited above) that, in some languages, verbs develop earlier than in languages such as English and other European languages and so the noun bias may be diminished or non-existent. Characteristics of the input to young children from caregivers seem to account for these differences. Where this is the case, care needs to be taken to sample early verbs as well as early nouns.

Simple sentences

In simple sentences words are combined to express propositions that go beyond simple identification or naming. Grammatically they contain minimally one verb. Verbs may be absent in early sentences, but sooner or later the child acquires the conventions for constructing a sentence around a verb. Arguments expressing thematic roles such as agent, patient, benefactive, locative, etc. will also minimally be present, but these may be implied and recoverable from the pragmatic context. Thematic roles may be expressed explicitly through noun phrases or prepositional phrases, as in English, or by means of inflection on the verb. Languages may rely on word order to make clear the thematic roles played by each element (so *John is hitting Mary* has a different meaning from *Mary is hitting John*), or word order may be comparatively free, with identification of thematic roles through grammatical inflections or case endings on nouns, determiners and/or prepositions. All of these possibilities have implications for the development of simple sentences and potentially facilitate or inhibit early acquisition. In *pro*-drop languages (e.g. Italian), subject pronouns are frequently omitted from sentences, with the verb inflection indicating who or what is carrying out the action. In some languages, 'radical *pro*-drop' occurs, with the omission of a range of sentence elements, whose reference is presumably recoverable from the context.

Spontaneous language samples may give an idea of the child's ability to get across the sort of information conveyed by simple sentences, but the implications for the acquisition of these different possibilities require further research. Relevant questions include, for example, whether sentences where *pro*-drop occurs are produced earlier than those where the subject of the verb must be expressed, albeit with a pronoun, and whether it takes longer to get to grips with sentence structures involving case endings than with those dependent on word order. Where formal testing is developed, or where an existing procedure is adapted to another language, contrasts may have to be explored carefully. In the *NRDLS* Comprehension Scale, for example, reversible active sentences are used (where either of two noun phrases could be the agent of the action) and the child has to demonstrate knowledge of English word-order rules in order to respond correctly. In languages where the word order is freer, the key cues could be provided by case endings (e.g. Latvian); however, there may be word orders that occur more commonly and thus are more readily comprehended by the child. A decision will need to be made about how much word order is varied across items, as well as ensuring that the important case contrasts are also represented.

With children who are bilingual, a further possible complication is that intra-sentential code-switching may occur once the child has moved beyond the one word stage in the production of language. Pert and Letts (2006) report on the use of a sentence elicitation measure (asking the child to describe simple pictures) to gain information about a child's simple sentence construction in Mirpuri. The task was administered by a Mirpuri-speaking bilingual co-worker, but nevertheless typically developing children all produced some code-switched utterances in their responses. Examples include the following:

(1)   Target picture:
      A man is throwing a ball

      Child's sentence:
      DADDY FOOTBALL *sat   -an   laga*
      Daddy   football   throw -will about to
      'daddy about to throw (the) ball.'

(2)   Target picture:
      A man drying his hands

      Child's sentence:
      DADDY *tolija   nal   at*   WASH *kar -na*   *pija*
      Daddy   towel with hands wash   do -ing + MALE is + MALE
      'Daddy is doing washing (his) hands with (a) towel.' (Pert & Letts, 2006: 364, 366)

The original intention was to produce an assessment procedure that could be used in one language, and then an equivalent version to be used in the child's other language. The idea of using each language independently in this context (and therefore being able to test each language independently using a common set of materials) proved, however, to be too simplistic. It appeared that code-switched forms were used routinely throughout the child's community and therefore any assessment of language production had to take this into account. Furthermore, the children demonstrated sophisticated grammatical abilities in integrating English verbs into their code-switched utterances in such a way that subject–verb agreement patterns were not violated. Issues of this sort that arise when assessing bilingual children are discussed further below.

Complex sentences

Sentences described as *complex* usually involve one of two features. First, canonical word order for simple sentences may be changed, as in questions and passive forms for English. These types of sentence are sometimes described as involving *movement*. For example, in the question, 'Who did Tom criticize?', the object of the verb moves from the postverbal position ('Tom criticized Fred') to the front of the clause. Passive structures in English involve the object of the verb moving to the preverbal position (e.g. 'Fred was criticized by Tom').

Second, one sentence (or clause) may be 'embedded' within another, as with subordinate clauses or relative clauses, e.g. 'Tom criticized Fred because he was rude' (subordinate clause beginning with *because*); 'Tom criticized the man who was rude' (relative clause modifying *the man*). Of course, complex sentences can also involve combinations of both of these features, as when a clause in the passive voice is embedded within a main clause, e.g. 'Tom felt sorry for the man who was bitten by a dog'. Generally, the processing load involved to comprehend or produce complex sentences is considered to be greater than that required for simple sentences, and this type of structure is generally acquired later. Several studies have also found that complex sentences are difficult for children with LI (for example, Friedmann & Novogrodsky, 2004; Novogrodsky & Friedmann, 2006; Stavrakaki, 2001; Van der Lely & Battell, 2003; van der Lely *et al.*, 2010).

Assessment for complex sentences can pose problems in terms of setting up items that will examine comprehension or elicit forms in production. Picture selection can work well for relative clauses, since they function to define noun phrases within a sentence more precisely (for example, the child can be asked to choose a picture that goes with *The man who is wearing a hat is running*, or *The dog is chasing the cat that has a white foot*) (see Gathercole *et al.*, 2013). For production, sentence repetition and modelling tasks can be useful (*NRDLS* uses a modelling procedure for eliciting relative clauses), and role-play can be used, for example, to elicit questions (e.g. the child is asked to role play a character who is trying to find things out by asking questions).

As with other structures, ways in which complex sentences are formed in different languages will vary. For example, the position of the *WH* word in *wh*-questions may vary (Dryer, 2008), which in turn will have implications for whether movement is involved. A variety of 'strategies' are described by Comrie and Katava (2008) for forming relative clauses, including case-marked relative pronouns and repetition of the main clause noun phrase. Positioning of relative clauses in relation to the noun phrase can also vary

(Flynn *et al.*, 2005). Importantly, passives, which in languages such as English are frequently tested as representative of later language development, are not present in many languages (Siewierska [2008] gives 211 languages without passive forms out of a total of 373). In other languages, passives may occur but too infrequently to be likely to feature in informal child language.

These variations will have an influence on order of acquisition and may contribute to second-learner errors or unusual patterns in bilingual speakers.

Checking appropriateness of test items

The above paragraphs illustrate that, even if a basic developmental progression can be identified that applies to language acquisition for all languages, there may be variations in the timing and order of the surface manifestations of these stages: the single word stage may reflect a noun bias, or may be represented by verbs and nouns equally; the structures used in both simple and complex sentences (for example, verb morphology) may vary in terms of time of emergence and consolidation, again depending on characteristics of the language. Of course, individual languages may also contain structures that are unique to that language or language group (an example might be mutations in Welsh; see Ball & Müller [1992] for a description and Tallerman [2006] for a recent discussion of syntax), and for these, if acquisition research on these structures is absent, the developmental sequence can only be guessed at (Gathercole [2007] reports on acquisition of gender patterns as expressed through the Welsh soft mutation). So, while candidates may emerge for testing, reliable information on their acquisition may not be available until norming data have been collected and analysed. In the short term, though, a number of strategies are available to help in confirming whether a structure is 'important' and appropriate to use in formal testing. For one, a native-speaker adult informant who shares the linguistic and cultural background of the target group should ideally be used, and he or she can help confirm the appropriateness of the vocabulary and structures for children. Additionally, it may be possible to trial items on small numbers of typically developing children from the given background to gain some information as to what can be expected in terms of acquisition. Finally, in cases in which individual children are causing concern, asking adults from the community to compare aspects of their language with age peers may be helpful.

Testing bilinguals

For monolingual professionals, the immediate concern when assessing a bilingual child tends to be that of finding ways of working with an unknown language or languages, especially when good descriptions and developmental norms are not available. This very real concern tends to mask further issues arising because of the unique linguistic profiles associated with bilingual language acquisition. The possibility of apparent 'delay' in one or both of the child's languages when compared to monolingual norms has already been mentioned. In order to get a full picture, assessment that allows the child to demonstrate his/her skills in all the languages s/he speaks is essential. However, this still raises questions about how to go about this. For example, does testing take place on two completely separate occasions, once exclusively in one language and once exclusively in the other? Or is the child presented with one set of procedures and encouraged to respond in whichever language s/he feels comfortable with? When looking at production of language, Pert and Letts (2003) reported on testing children from a Pakistani heritage background using a simple picture description task. The pictures were presented by a bilingual co-worker and in this situation a number of interesting factors emerged. First, the children did not necessarily respond in the language reported to be their home language, but responded instead in a different Pakistani heritage language (often Mirpuri, considered by speakers to be a low-status language and which does not have a written form). Second, as mentioned, the children used high numbers of code-switched utterances in which English lexical forms were inserted into matrix Mirpuri sentences. Restricting the children's responses to a predefined language would have resulted in an underestimate of their linguistic development in these cases.

Testing comprehension raises obvious problems as the tester will need to know which language it is appropriate to use. It may be possible to give an item again in the child's other language if the child fails to respond (or fails to respond correctly) in one language. Here it will be necessary to take into account that the child will likely already have gained some insight regarding the nature of the item from the first presentation, even if s/he has not fully understood it at that point. Deciding how to proceed here would very much depend on the purpose of assessment; in the context of potential LI, an overview of the child's ability to communicate, regardless of language, is likely to be required.

Integration of Testing with Other Assessments and Conclusions

When using formal testing procedures with children it is important to remember that these procedures are tools only and that the right questions must be asked in the first place. If the question concerns the extent to which a child may be at risk for LI, then a test procedure may indicate potential linguistic areas of difficulty, and supply a comparison with other children in the form of norms. The tester must always be mindful of the appropriateness or not of these norms to the target child, and to the appropriateness of using a procedure of this type with the child. Carter et al. (2005) illustrate how the cultural and educational experiences of the child can strongly influence outcomes when formal test procedures are used. It is important to collect background information on the child and his or her context in order to take into account effects of this kind.

The formal test should never be the only assessment procedure used. The child's overall general ability to communicate, however this is done, is important, as is his/her use of language in spontaneous situations when not constrained by the testing situation. Above all, comparison must be made with a relevant peer group of children sharing the same linguistic background and experiences. Where such a peer group is not available, it is important to proceed with caution.

It can be seen that assessment of early comprehension and production of spoken language in a bilingual context is not straightforward. Lack of knowledge of acquisition norms for particular languages and for bilingual acquisition of these languages makes this particularly problematic. Nevertheless, there are strategies that the professional can use, and knowledge in this area is developing and is the focus of much current research interest.

Summary: Important Issues When Assessing the Language of Bilingual Children

- Being bilingual does not increase a child's risk for LI, but bilingual children are as much at risk as the monolingual population.
- In developing assessment procedures for use with bilingual children, finding appropriate peer groups for comparison is of crucial importance, but may be difficult.
- Direct comparison with monolingual norms for particular structures in a particular language is not appropriate.
- It may be normal for a bilingual child to use extensive intra-sentential code-switching.
- Typical features of SLA may look similar to those associated with SLI, but do not necessarily imply LI in L2 children.
- Formal test results should always be complemented by other measures.
- There is evidence for the effectiveness of intervention for language at an early age, but conclusive markers that indicate impairment may not be apparent early enough to distinguish typically developing from LI children.
- A number of factors should be taken into account when developing assessment procedures in a range of languages:
  - presence or absence of a noun bias in early words;
  - ways in which thematic role assignment is realized grammatically (e.g. word order/inflections);
  - whether pro-drop is a normal feature of the language;

- ways in which *wh*-questions and relative clauses are formed;
- structures that may be absent from a language (e.g. tense, passives) or unique to only a small number of languages.
- It may be useful to elicit information from adult informants who speak the relevant languages, and/or to recruit some of a child's peers for comparison purposes.
- The child's cultural background and experience must always be considered when making an assessment.

Acknowledgements

The ideas presented in this chapter have been heavily influenced by experience working on the *New Reynell Developmental Language Scales (NRDLS)* and the *Multilingual Toolkit* that accompanies the Scales. I am therefore indebted to Dr Indra Sinka for her collaborative work on the toolkit and to both Indra and Professor Susan Edwards for the major data collection exercise and subsequent discussions that culminated in the production of *NRDLS*.

References

Archibald, L.M.D. and Gathercole, S.E. (2006) Short-term and working memory in specific language impairment. *International Journal of Language and Communication Disorders* 41, 675–694.

Ball, M. and Müller, N. (1992) *Mutation in Welsh*. London: Routledge.

Bedore, L. and Leonard, L. (2005) Grammatical morphology deficits in Spanish-speaking children with specific language impairment. *Journal of Speech, Language and Hearing Research* 44, 905–924.

Bercow, J. (2008) *The Bercow Report: A Review of Services for Children and Young People (0–19) with Speech, Language and Communication Needs*. https://www.education.gov.uk/publications/standard/publicationdetail/page1/DCSF-00632-2008

Berko-Gleason, J. and Ratner, N.B. (2009) *The Development of Language* (7th edn). Boston, MA: Pearson.

Bialystok, E. (1991) Metalinguistic dimensions of bilingual language proficiency. In E. Bialystok (ed.) *Language Processing in Bilingual Children* (pp. 113–140). Cambridge: Cambridge University Press.

Bortolini, U., Caselli, M.C., Deevy, P. and Leonard, L.B. (2002) Specific language impairment in Italian: The first steps in the search for a clinical marker. *International Journal of Language and Communication Disorders* 37, 77–93.

Cable, A.L. and Domsch, C. (2011) Systematic review of the literature on the treatment of children with late language emergence. *International Journal of Language and Communication Disorders* 46, 138–154.

Carrow, E. (1973) *Test of Auditory Comprehension of Language: English/Spanish*. Austin, TX: Learning Concepts.

Carter, J.A., Lees, J.A., Murira, G.M., Gona, J., Neville, B.G.R. and Newton, C.R.J.C. (2005) Issues in the development of cross-cultural assessments of speech and language for children. *International Journal of Language and Communication Disorders* 37, 77–93.

Chiat, S. and Roy, P. (2007) The Preschool Repetition Test: An evaluation of performance in typically developing and clinically referred children. *Journal of Speech, Language and Hearing Research* 50, 429–443.

CHILDES (2003) Child Language Data Exchange System website. http://childes.psy.cmu. edu.

Choi, S. and Gopnik, A. (1995) Early acquisition of verbs in Korean: A cross-linguistic study. *Journal of Child Language* 22, 497–529.

Comrie, B. and Kuteva, T. (2008) Relativization strategies. In M. Haspelmath, M. Dryer, D. Gil and B. Comrie (eds) *The World Atlas of Language Structures Online*. Munich: Max Planck Digital Library. http://wals.info/supplement/8.

Crystal, D., Fletcher, P. and Garman, M. (1976) *Linguistic Assessment, Remediation and Screening Procedure (LARSP)*. London: Edward Arnold.

Cupples, R.B. (2011) Assessment of child language disorders. In R.B. Hoodin (ed.) *Intervention in Child Language Disorders* (pp. 33–44). London: Jones & Bartlett.

Dabrowska, E. (2004) *Language, Mind and Brain*. Edinburgh: Edinburgh University Press.

de Jong, J., Çavus, N. and Baker, A. (2010) Language impairment in Turkish–Dutch bilingual children. In S. Topbas and M. Yavas (eds) *Communication Disorders in Turkish in Monolingual and Multilingual Settings* (pp. 288–300). Bristol: Multilingual Matters.

Dromi, E., Leonard, L.B., Adam, G. and Zadunaisky-Erlich, S. (1999) Verb agreement morphology in Hebrew-speaking children with specific language impairment. *Journal of Speech, Language and Hearing Research* 42, 1414–1431.

Dryer, M.S. (2008) Position of interrogative phrases in content questions. In M. Haspelmath, M. Dryer, D. Gil and B. Comrie (eds) *The World Atlas of Language Structures Online*. Munich: Max Planck Digital Library. http://wals.info/feature/93.

Duncan, D., Gibbs, D., Noor, N.S. and Whittaker, H.M. (1988) *Sandwell Bilingual Screening Assessment Scales for Expressive Punjabi and English*. Windsor: NFER-Nelson.

Edwards, S., Fletcher, P., Garman, M., Hughes, A., Letts, C. and Sinka, I. (1997) *The Reynell Developmental Language Scales III: The University of Reading Edition*. London: NFER-Nelson.

Edwards, S., Letts, C. and Sinka, I. (2011) *The New Reynell Developmental Language Scales*. London: GL-Assessment.

Flynn, S., Foley, C. and Vinnitskaya, I. (2005) New paradigm for the study of simultaneous v. sequential bilingualism. In J. Cohen, K. McAlister, K. Rolstad and J. MacSwan (eds) *ISB4: Proceedings of the 4th International Symposium on Bilingualism* (pp. 768–774). Somerville, MA: Cascadilla Press.

Friedmann, N. and Novogrodsky, R. (2004) The acquisition of relative clause comprehension in Hebrew: A study of SLI and normal development. *Journal of Child Language* 31, 661–681.

Gathercole, V.C.M. (2007) Miami and North Wales, so far and yet so near: A constructivist account of morphosyntactic development in bilingual children. *International Journal of Bilingual Education and Bilingualism* 10, 224–247.

Gathercole, V.C.M. and Thomas, E.M. (2009) Bilingual first-language development: Dominant language takeover, threatened minority language take-up. *Bilingualism: Language and Cognition* 12, 213–237.

Gathercole, V.C.M., Thomas, E.M. and Hughes, E. (2008) Designing a normed receptive vocabulary test for bilingual populations: A model from Welsh. *International Journal of Bilingual Education and Bilingualism* 11, 678–720.

Gathercole, V.C.M., Thomas, E.M., Roberts, E., Hughes, C. and Hughes, E.K. (2013) Why assessment needs to take exposure into account: Vocabulary and grammatical abilities in bilingual children. In V.C.M. Gathercole (ed.) *Issues in the Assessment of Bilinguals* (pp. 20–55). Bristol: Multilingual Matters.

Gatt, D., Letts C.A. and Klee T. (2008) Lexical mixing in the early productive vocabularies of Maltese children: Implications for intervention. *Clinical Linguistics & Phonetics* 22, 267–274.

Hansson, K. and Leonard, L.B. (2003) The use and productivity of verb morphology in specific language impairment: An examination of Swedish. *Linguistics* 41, 351–379.

Hoff, E. (2005) *Language Development* (3rd edn). Belmont, CA: Wadsworth.

Hoff, E., Core, C., Place, S. Rumiche, R., Senor, M. and Parra, M. (2012) Dual language exposure and early bilingual development. *Journal of Child Language* 39, 1–27.

Hulit, L.M. and Howard, H.R. (2005) *Born to Talk: An Introduction to Speech and Language Development* (4th edn). London: Allyn & Bacon.

Isaac, K. (2002) *Speech Pathology and Linguistic Diversity.* London: Wiley.

Kim, M., McGregor, K.K. and Thompson, C.K. (2000) Early lexical development in English- and Korean-speaking children: Language-general and language-specific patterns. *Journal of Child Language* 27, 225–270.

Kunnari, S., Savinainen-Makkonen, T., Leonard, L.B., Makinen, L., Tolonen, A.K., Luotonen, M. and Leinonen, E. (2011) Children with specific language impairment in Finnish: The use of tense and agreement inflections. *Journal of Child Language* 38, 999–1027.

Law, J., Boyle, J., Harris, F., Harkness, A. and Nye, C. (2000) Prevalence and natural history of primary speech and language delay: Findings from a systematic review of the literature. *International Journal of Language and Communication Disorders* 35, 165–188.

Leonard, L.B. (1998) *Children with Specific Language Impairment.* Cambridge, MA: MIT Press.

Leonard, L.B., Wong, A., Deevy, P., Stokes, S. and Fletcher, P. (2006) The production of passives by children with specific language impairment acquiring English and Cantonese. *Applied Psycholinguistics* 27, 267–299.

Letts, C. and Sinka, I. (2011) *Multilingual Toolkit.* London: GL-Assessment.

Lidz, C.S. (2003) *Early Childhood Assessment.* Hoboken, NJ: Wiley.

Lindsay, G., Dockrell, J., Desforges, M., Law, J. and Peacey, N. (2010) Meeting the needs of children and young people with speech, language and communication difficulties. *International Journal of Language and Communication Disorders* 45, 448–460.

Malvern, D. and Richards, B. (2002) Investigating accommodation in language proficiency interviews using a new measure of lexical diversity. *Language Testing* 19, 85–104.

McArthur–Bates CDI (2003) McArthur–Bates Communicative Development Inventories website. http://www.sci.sdsu.edu/cdi/adaptations_ol.htm.

Novadgradsky, R. and Friedmann, N. (2006) The production of relative clauses in syntactic SLI: A window to the nature of impairment. *Advances in Speech-Language Pathology* 8, 364–375.

Orgassa, A. (2009) Specific language impairment in a bilingual context: The acquisition of Dutch by Turkish–Dutch learners. LOT Dissertation No. 220. University of Amsterdam, Utrecht.

Paradis, J. (2010) Bilingual children's acquisition of English verb morphology: Effects of language exposure, structure complexity, and task type. *Language Learning* 60, 651–680.

Paradis, J., Nicoladis, E. and Genesee, F. (2000) Early emergence of structural constraints on code mixing. *Bilingualism: Language and Cognition* 3, 245–261.

Patterson, J.L. (1998) Expressive vocabulary development and word combinations of Spanish–English bilingual toddlers. *American Journal of Speech-language Pathology* 7, 46–56.

Peña, E.D., Bedore, L.M. and Zlatic-Giunta, R. (2002) Category-generation performance of bilingual children: The influence of condition, category and language. *Journal of Speech, Language and Hearing Research* 45, 938–947.

Pert, S. and Letts, C. (2003) Developing an expressive language assessment for children in Rochdale with a Pakistani heritage background. *Child Language Teaching and Therapy* 19, 267–289.

Pert, S. and Letts, C. (2006) Codeswitching in Mirpuri-speaking Pakistani heritage pre-school children: Bilingual language acquisition. *International Journal of Bilingualism* 10, 349–374.

Reynell, J. (1977) *The Reynell Developmental Language Scales: Revised Edition.* London: NFER.

Rice, M. (2003) A unified model of specific and general language delay: Grammatical tense as a clinical marker. In Y. Levy and J. Schaeffer (eds) *Language Competence Across Populations* (pp. 63–94). Hillsdale, NJ: Lawrence Erlbaum.

Riches, N.G., Loucas, T., Baird, G., Charman, T. and Siminoff, E. (2010) Sentence repetition in adolescents with specific language impairment and autism: An investigation of complex syntax. *International Journal of Language and Communication Disorders* 45, 47–60.

Roberts, S.S. and Leonard, L.B. (1997) Grammatical deficits in German and English: A crosslinguistic study of children with specific language impairment. *First Language* 17, 131–150.

Sierwierska, A. (2008) Passive constructions. In M. Haspelmath, M. Dryer, D. Gil and B. Comrie (eds) *The World Atlas of Language Structures Online.* Munich: Max Planck Digital Library. http://wals.info/feature/107.

Stavrakaki, S. (2001) Comprehension of reversible relative clauses in specifically language impaired and normally developing Greek children. *Brain and Language* 77, 419–431.

Stavrakaki, S. and Van der Lely, H. (2010) Production and comprehension of pronouns by Greek children with specific language impairment. *British Journal of Developmental Psychology* 28, 189–216.

Tallerman, E. (2006) The syntax of Welsh 'direct object mutation' revisited. *Lingua* 116, 1750–1776.

Thordardottir, E. (2008) Language-specific effects of task demands on the manifestation of specific language impairment: A comparison of English and Icelandic. *Journal of Speech, Language and Hearing Research* 51, 992–937.

Van der Lely, H. and Battell, J. (2003) Wh-movement in children with grammatical SLI: a test of the RDDR hypothesis. *Language* 79, 153–181.

Van der Lely, H., Jones, M. and Marshall, C.R. (2010) Who did Buzz see someone? Grammaticality judgements of wh-questions in typically developing children and children with grammatical SLI. *Lingua* 121, 408–422.

Van der Lely, H. and Stollwerck, L. (1997) Binding theory and specifically language impaired children. *Cognition* 62, 153–181.

4 Using Parental Report Assessment for Bilingual Preschoolers: The Basque Experience

Maria-José Ezeizabarrena, Julia Barnes, Iñaki García, Andoni Barreña and Margareta Almgren

In this chapter the structure of the Basque adaptation of the MacArthur–Bates CDI Tests is presented. The criteria and decisions adopted during the adaptation into a language with the complex characteristics of the Basque language are reported. Parental reports of over 2600 children between the ages of 8 months and 4 years 2 months were collected, including information on the production of communicative gestures, the comprehension and production of vocabulary, and the production of morphology and of morphosyntactically complex structures. The development observed across the different components of the instrument serve as a reference for the study of the steps typically developing children undergo, and the instrument permits the study of the effect of the degree of exposure to the language, a fundamental aspect in a bilingual community. Data analysed (a) suggest that the degree of exposure may affect differently the components under study, and (b) reveal that the effect of the degree of exposure is visible for the instrument from age 2 years 4 months, increasing to over 20% from age 3 years onwards.

Introduction

The MacArthur–Bates Communicative Development Inventories (CDI) were originally designed by Fenson *et al.* (1993) as a tool to measure the language development of infants and toddlers based on parental report. A further goal of that instrument was to detect developmental delay at very early ages (below 2 years 6 months), thus enabling remedial action to be taken. To date the Inventories have been adapted for over 40 different languages throughout the world. The reliability and validity of the instrument have been reported in Fenson *et al.* (1993) for American English, by Jackson-Maldonado *et al.* (2003) for Mexican Spanish, and by López Ornat *et al.* (2005) for European Spanish, among others.

The CDI-1 *Words and gestures* questionnaire, covering ages 8–15 months, focuses on the understanding and production of words and communicative gestures. The CDI-2 *Words and sentences*, covering 16–30 months, focuses on production, and the questionnaire includes a longer list of vocabulary items, a wider range of morphosyntactic categories, such as inflected nouns and verbs, as well as a list of linguistic structure-pairs attested in infants' spontaneous corpora at different developmental stages. Finally, the CDI-3 covers 31–40 months of age. Parents (in most cases) and primary caregivers are used as observers to complete these questionnaires, reflecting their child's growing proficiency, marking in one column the words their child understands at the time of filling in the questionnaire, in a separate column the gestures they produce (in CDI-1), and in another section the words and grammatical items the child produces (in CDI-2 and CDI-3).

The present chapter will describe the adaptation of the MacArthur–Bates CDI questionnaires (Fenson *et al.*, 1993, 2007) into Basque – henceforth the KGNZ (Komunikazio Garapenaren Neurketarako Zerrenda [List to measure communicative development]: the KGNZ-1 (8–15 months), KGNZ-2 (16–30 months) and KGNZ-3 (30–50 months), respectively. In addition, some of the issues entailed, and the results obtained so far in the research conducted by the KGNZ research team will be presented.

The data constitute the most extensive corpus of parental reports on Basque child language ever collected. They primarily measure the comprehension and production of Basque vocabulary and grammar in children exposed to the language by both parents from birth. However, as is to be expected in bilingual communities, data from children exposed to varying degrees of bilingual input from parents, grandparents, caretakers and other sources were inevitably gathered in the process.

The sociolinguistic context in the Basque Country

Basque has been a minority and minoritized language for centuries, and has been practically absent in official education until recently, although it was taught before (and even clandestinely during) the period of its repression under the regime of Franco from 1939 to 1975. It was not until after 1980 that a slow recovery began to take place, mainly through educational programmes initiated after Basque was recognized as one of the official regional languages in Spain by the Spanish Constitution of 1978. At present, Basque is spoken by about a million people living on either side of the Pyrenees Mountains, along the Atlantic Coast. Administratively, Basque speakers belong to several historical territories, or communities, located in two European states (Spain and France). On the French side, the three Basque provinces of Lapurdi, Behe-Nafarroa and Xuberoa constitute the *Département des Pyrénées Atlantiques*. On the Spanish side there are four provinces: one is Navarra, which is an autonomous administration (*Comunidad Foral de Navarra*) within the Spanish state, and the three other provinces are Bizkaia, Gipuzkoa and Araba, which form the Basque Autonomous Community (*Comunidad Autónoma del País Vasco*). The Basque Autonomous Community is the most densely populated area and the one in which Basque is spoken the most, and it is where most of our data were collected.

The society is officially bilingual in the Basque Autonomous Community and in the northern part of Navarra, requiring, for example, that administrative and legal texts be published in both official languages and labelling and signposting be bilingual in Spanish and Basque. However, the official use of Basque does not occur to the same extent in the rest of Navarra and in the French provinces, where Basque does not have official status. Despite the existence of a daily newspaper, some radio channels and a television channel in Basque – the latter mostly restricted to the Basque Autonomous Community – the media (press, radio, TV) are still predominantly in Spanish or French throughout the seven provinces described.

The number of Basque speakers varies across the three major communities, and also within each community. Most small rural areas in Gipuzkoa, Bizkaia and the northern part of Navarra on the Spanish side are traditionally Basque speaking, as the language has been transmitted orally. This is also true for the interior of the French Basque Country. However, on the coast as well as in the capitals of the Basque Autonomous Community, the percentage of native speakers is lower. Most adult speakers over 40 years of age, especially those from older generations, attended school in Spanish or French, which means that all native speakers of Basque from those generations became Basque–Spanish or Basque–French bilinguals. However, not all adult speakers of Spanish or French in the Basque Country are bilingual, resulting in a sort of asymmetric social bilingualism. Official reports from 2006 indicate that 58.9% out of the 2,500,000 inhabitants older than 16 years are monolingual speakers of Spanish or French, whereas 41.1% are Spanish–Basque or French–Basque bilinguals. Only 25.7% of the bilinguals use both languages fluently and 15.4% are receptive bilinguals, who understand Basque but have only a basic productive level (Eusko Jaurlaritza, 2006). The rate of bilinguals reported in the Basque Autonomous Community in 2006 was higher (54.9% or 37.48% fluent + 17.34% receptive bilinguals) than the general rate reported for the whole Basque Country. In fact, there are

1,105,331 Basque speakers out of 2,016,257 inhabitants older than 5 years in the Basque Autonomous Community, although rates of knowledge of Basque vary across the three provinces from 43% in Araba to 70% in Gipuzkoa (Eusko Jaurlaritza, 2009).

Naturalistic language transmission, e.g. in the home, is generally considered one of the most important factors in language survival. Official reports indicate that Basque is the first language for only about 20% of the population found across the territories that constitute the Basque Country. Thus statistical data from 2001 published by the Basque Institute of Statistics (2004) show that the majority of the population of the Basque Autonomous Community (74%) had Spanish as their mother tongue, 22% had Basque as their mother tongue and only a few (4%) had both Spanish and Basque as native languages. Five years later these rates were very similar, as 76.2% had Spanish, 18.7% Basque and 5.1% had both Spanish and Basque as native languages in this community (Eusko Jaurlaritza, 2009). Moreover, these rates do not differ greatly from the general data for the Basque Country obtained in 2006, when 78.7% had Spanish or French as first language, 16.5% Basque and 4.8% two languages, Basque and Spanish or Basque and French (Eusko Jaurlaritza, 2009). See Figure 4.1 for a more detailed distribution across the three provinces of the Basque Autonomous Community.

The apparent disagreement between the mean rates of the population having Basque as (one of) the first language(s) acquired (around 20%) and rates of around 40% of (bilingual) users of Basque cannot be explained in terms of

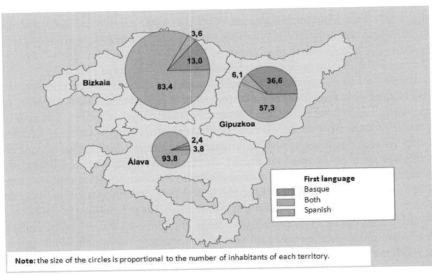

Note: the size of the circles is proportional to the number of inhabitants of each territory.

Figure 4.1 First language of the population in the Basque Autonomous Community in 2006 (Eusko Jaurlaritza, 2009)

naturalistic language transmission alone and requires some more extended explanation. Data show that most Basque speakers grew up in families in which at least one of the parents was a Basque speaker, but not all bilinguals are descendants of Basque-speaking parents. In fact, only 70% of bilinguals older than 16 years are reported to be descendants of (one or two) Basque-speaking parents in the Basque Autonomous Community, indicating that 30% of Basque speakers in this group have learnt the language outside the parental environment and became Spanish–Basque bilinguals through the educational system. The rate of 45.2% monolingual (5 years of age or older) Spanish speakers in this area in 2006 contrasts with the 65.9% of monolingual Spanish speakers 15 years earlier. The transformation is mostly visible in the youngest age groups. In 1991 rates of monolinguals were consistently higher than 60% in all age groups. By 2006, these rates persisted only in the oldest age groups (over 50 years), whereas the rates decreased to between 30% and 55% between 30 and 50 years of age, and decreased still further to rates below 20% in the youngest group, between 5 and 25 years of age (Eusko Jaurlaritza, 2009).

Such a decrease in monolinguals is a consequence of the increase in fluent and receptive bilinguals and is just a small sample of the more general socio-linguistic transformation observed in this region during the last three decades. The numbers of young and adult monolingual Spanish speakers under 40 years of age have decreased considerably thanks to the intensive and extensive Basque teaching programmes developed within the regular educational system for children and in outside curricular programmes for adults. Noticeably, in 2006 the number of monolingual Spanish speakers in the Basque Autonomous Community was 137,300 lower than in 1991.

Recent official reports indicate that 90% of 2-year old children and 100% of those aged 3 years or older in the Basque Autonomous Community are enrolled in the school system (Eustat, 2011). The structural organization of the Basque educational system contains a first block of non-compulsory infant education (0–6 years) divided into two blocks: 0–3 and 4–6 years. This education takes place mostly in Basque, although there are some bilingual or even trilingual Kindergartens in which Basque, Spanish and a foreign language are used daily. More than 90% of the students in the Basque Autonomous Community attend Basque immersion (or maintenance) programmes developed for compulsory primary (6–12 years) and secondary education (12–16 years): 60.5% are in Basque Immersion and 30.1% are in Basque Middle Immersion models (ISEI-IVEI, 2010). It should also be pointed out that in the Basque Autonomous Community a segment of the adult population has attended highly intensive language and literacy programmes in Basque (see Figure 4.2). As an example, in 1978 only 5% of the teachers were trained to teach in Basque, and by 2005 this percentage had risen to 70%.

A further consideration in the Basque sociolinguistic situation is the linguistic distance between the languages in contact. From a linguistic point of view, Basque is an isolated language, which means that it is not genetically

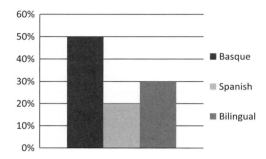

Figure 4.2 Language distribution in primary and secondary education in the Basque Autonomous Community

related to any Indo-European (or non-Indo-European) language. Typologically, it is an ergative language, with agglutinative morphology and an SOV syntactic word order, in contrast to the surrounding Romance languages Spanish and French, which are accusative, fusional languages and have SVO word order. Basque has a very rich verbal and nominal morphology (although no morphological gender system in the nominal domain) and marks case and number postpositionally. Aspect marking is suffixed to the main verb, and it is the auxiliary that marks tense. The intransitive and transitive verb systems, inflected for subject, direct object and indirect object agreement, are quite complex. Hence, it greatly differs from the Romance languages with which it is in contact, as they are prepositional and encode person-marking on the verb for subject agreement only.[1]

The KGNZ Study

Our goal was to develop a valid battery of CDI measures for Basque. Our questionnaires thus focused initially on measuring native monolingual development during the first stages of language use. The fact that the questionnaire was written in Basque, a language very different from the Romance languages with which it is in contact, influenced the kind of parental units that could be involved with data collection using the KGNZ questionnaires. Parents (at least one of them) needed to be Basque speakers and able to read the documents in that language. Consequently, the vast majority of data collected corresponded to children growing up in monolingual Basque or in bilingual Basque–Spanish or Basque–French families in which at least one of the parents has a fairly high level of Basque knowledge.

It should be noted that, even though the initial aim of the data collectors was to focus on monolingual subjects, the study also includes different degrees of bilinguals in the sample. Taking into account that children of our study are acquiring a minority language within a (partially) bilingual society, during the data collection for the KGNZs, special care was taken that parents and caregivers reported on the amounts of Basque and Spanish/French and other languages the children were exposed to. In addition, they reported on language use between the parents, and a section for this purpose was included on the last page of the questionnaires.

In the following sections, we will explain in detail how the KGNZ, the Basque CDI, was constructed and how the data were obtained, followed by a description of the general findings from the overall data, and then an exploration of the effects of exposure to Basque on children's performance.

Adaptation of the English CDI into Basque

Method

The KGNZ research group was comprised of scholars working in different universities and with wide and diverse experience in the study of bilingualism. A varied spectrum of perspectives comprised the team's experience from the beginning, including expertise in preschool, primary and secondary education, the early acquisition of grammar in monolingual and bilingual settings, the dialectology of the Basque language, and the statistical treatment of psycho-sociolinguistic data. Its members came from the University of Mondragon, the University of the Basque Country, the University of Salamanca, the Universidad Pública de Navarra and Seaska.

Work on the KGNZ was initiated in 2000. The design of the final version of the KGNZ-1 and KGNZ-2 lasted around two years, followed by extensive piloting and then data collection, which was completed in 2006. During this period data were shared with the linguistic community in partial papers (Arratibel *et al.*, 2005; Barreña, Ezeizabarrena, & Garcia, 2008; Barreña, Garcia, Ezeizabarrena *et al.*, 2008; García *et al.*, 2005), which preceded the manual written in Basque and published as Barreña, Garcia *et al.* (2008). The manual contained the main results obtained from a sample containing 1417 valid questionnaires, 442 corresponding to 8–15 months of age (KGNZ-1) and 975 to 16–30 months of age (KGNZ-2). This manual followed very closely the structure and contents of the original that was produced by Fenson *et al.* (1993), including the statistical analysis, tables of percentiles for all the sections of the questionnaires, and measurements of reliability and validity of the instruments.

The two Basque questionnaires follow the original American English CDI-1 *Words and gestures* and CDI-2 *Words and sentences* closely, organized into two sections (plus a socio-biolinguistic section): lexical (396 items) and gesture (63 items) sections in CDI-1, and lexical (680 items) and grammar (111 items) sections in CDI-2. Item numbers in KGNZ diverge only slightly from the original in the lexical part. In contrast, substantial differences can be observed in the grammar section, due to the typological differences between the English and Basque grammars, especially in relation to degree of morphological complexity. The lexical sections in both questionnaires are divided into semantic fields and the vocabulary items also follow the original American version, although some items that had too strong a cultural bias (e.g. *pancake, fire truck, porch*) were deleted or replaced by items that were thought to be closer to Basque small children's reality (e.g. *tortilla*, 'omelette'; *anbulantzia*, 'ambulance', *balkoi*, 'balcony'). The gesture section in CDI-1 is divided into five sections, as is the grammar section in CDI-2, in addition to the section in which parents are asked to write down the three longest sentences produced recently by the child in order to estimate mean length of utterances produced by the child (MaxLU).

The KGNZ-1 *Hitzak eta Keinuak* [*Words and gestures*] questionnaire (8–15 months) focuses on the understanding and production of 397 items along the 19 semantic fields of the vocabulary checklist section and the production of 63 communicative gestures. Parents are asked to mark in one column the words their child understands and in a separate column the words the child understands and produces. In the presentation of data that follows, we will pay special attention to data from the sections in KGNZ-1 on: sounds; games and routines; nouns related to persons, objects, animals, etc.; action words or verbs; and descriptive words or adjectives. These are the most frequent categories in young children's vocabularies and constitute the main body of the questionnaire in most languages available so far. Other categories referring to quantifiers, pronouns, adverbs, etc. are less frequent.

The KGNZ-2 *Hitzak eta esaldiak* [*Words and sentences*], covering ages 16–30 months, contains 654 items in 21 categories in its vocabulary checklist section and 84 items in the grammar section (46 morphological items and 37 questions about sentence complexity).

The adaptation into Basque was not straightforward due to the variation, mostly observed in vocabulary, across the many dialects spoken in the seven provinces spread over Spain and France. Furthermore, as the standardized variety of Basque called *Batua* [unified] has been learned as a second language by some parents, this variety is used by them with their children, adding an additional variety with less local specificity. In order to reflect this diversity, experts and informants representing the dialectal varieties were involved in the creation of the tool in order to make the KGNZ as representative as possible of the language used in speech to children and easily understandable to the Basque-speaking parents who would be using it. For this reason, two or even three lexical options were made available for some of the items of vocabulary, ordered from the most to least extended option. Such variability contrasts with the original and other versions of the CDI. In contrast, no such plurality was necessary for the gesture and grammar sections, as morphological items and alternates show fewer dialectal variations in this language.

A further issue was that of Basque's complex agglutinative morphology, which contrasts with the scarce inflectional morphology of English. Basque is an ergative language that exhibits 16 morphological cases in the nominal domain and a very rich morphology of person and tense on the verb. Verbs agree with their subjects, direct objects and indirect objects, and all three person markings may be expressed overtly or by zero morphemes. Moreover, Basque allows null arguments and its head-final nature makes articles, auxiliaries, postpositions and complementisers appear (suffixed) after the elements they would introduce in head-initial languages like English, Spanish or French. Thus, the existence of a lower number of words in the Basque sentence when compared to English is compensated for with a higher number of morphological units in each word. Consequently, measurements of utterance length (MaxLU) in the original and in the adaptation languages become more or less comparable, depending on the unit (morphemes/words) taken for measurement.

Finally, in the socio-biolinguistic section, unlike in other CDIs from monolingual contexts, parents are asked for some additional information such as the number of family members, the number of hours a week each member of the family spends talking with the child, and in which language, in both KGNZ-1 and -2.

The KGNZ-3, the third component of the Basque CDI-instrument, is a follow-up of the preceding KGNZ-1 and KGNZ-2, just as the original CDI-3 was the next step after the English CDI-1 and CDI-2. Similar to its predecessor, the CDI-2, the CDI-3 was designed primarily for the study of the production of vocabulary and grammar by children older than 30 months of age. This third questionnaire has some specific properties that distinguish it from the previous two in the original version in American English. The greatest difference between CDI-3 and its predecessors is its length, which is only a couple of pages, making the time needed to fill it in much shorter (about 20 minutes) for the parents. Data are therefore collected more easily. Unlike the previous two questionnaires, the CDI-3 has been adapted to very few languages. To our knowledge, only the Mexican Spanish version and the Basque version have been completed so far, and results obtained on both have been recently presented to the international community (Ezeizabarrena et al., 2011; Jackson-Maldonado, 2011).

CDI-3 is much shorter than the previous two because of the reduced item list contained in the vocabulary section ($N = 100$) in comparison to the vocabulary lists with over 350 words included in each of CDI-1 and CDI-2. CDI-3 and KGNZ-3 both include two more sections, which are designed in question format, one referring to grammatical structures (12 items in the CDI-1) and the other called *Use of language*, containing questions intended to assess children's knowledge (comprehension) of some logical and mathematical terms (12 questions).

The items selected for inclusion in the KGNZ-3 correspond to the following categories: vocabulary items like nouns and non-inflected verbs in the vocabulary section; questions about the use of suffixes corresponding to nominal inflection of case and postpositions; a series of present tense intransitive and transitive auxiliaries, some of them inflected for present tense subject agreement, subject-direct object agreement, subject-indirect object agreement, or subject-direct object-indirect object agreement, and some of them in relation to past tense. See Table 4.1 for a more detailed comparison between the structure of KGNZ-3 and the original CDI-3.

Although the Basque KGNZ-3 contains the same sections as the original CDI-3, there are noticeable qualitative and quantitative differences, mostly motivated by the specific morphosyntactic properties of the language and/or by the methodological decisions adopted by the team during its development. One of the differences is that the age range of children reported varies considerably between the CDI-3 (30–40 months) and the Basque KGNZ-3 (30–50 months). The main reason for this was that the ceiling effects observed in the English version of CDI-2 (before 30) and CDI-3 (before 40) were not observed in the age-paired groups studied with the Basque versions KGNZ-2 and KGNZ-3.

The adaptation of the CDI-3 into Basque took from 2008 to 2011. Different pilot tests and versions preceded the design of the final version of the KGNZ-3 in 2010. Following Fenson et al.'s (1993) initial proposal that the CDI instrument should be adapted, not translated, into the target languages, and in the absence of adaptations to other languages that could be used as a model, the KGNZ group established a procedure for determining which and how many items should be included in the final version. As a general rule, some items of the original version were translated and included, as well as a selection of items from the KGNZ-1 and KGNZ-2 (Barreña, Garcia et al., 2008) that were considered 'informative' enough for the study. The less informative items were discarded. Such less informative items included items that did not allow for discrimination in the age groups under study (30–50 months) because of being either too easy for most children across age

Table 4.1 Structural specificities of the CDI-3 and the Basque KGNZ-3

	CDI-3 (128 items)	KGNZ-3 (199 items + socio-biolinguistic data)
Expressive vocabulary	100 items	120 items
Grammar		
• Morphology	—	16 suffixes + 20 inflected verb forms
• Word combination	1 question	1 question
• Sentence complexity	12 structure pairs	29 structure pairs
• Using language	12 questions	10 questions
• Longest sentences	3 items	3 items
Socio-biolinguistic data	—	22 items

groups (*ceiling* effects) or too difficult for most of them (*plateau* effects), or because they did not belong to the children's cultural environment. For instance, some words like *dinosaurioa* 'dinosaur' were simply translated from the original English, whereas words like *cowboy* were not included in the adaptation, as they are unknown to most Basque children; in contrast, words like *gezurra* 'lying' or *fantasma/mamua* 'ghost' were included in the Basque version in spite of not existing in the English CDI-3. Many new lexical items included in the first section, as well as many grammatical items included in the second one, had been reported in previous longitudinal studies to occur in children's spontaneous productions (e.g. Almgren, 2002; Barreña, 1995; Elosegi, 1998; Ezeizabarrena, 1996, 2003; Zubiri, 1997).

In relation to production, for which parents are asked to mark the items their child produces, KGNZ-3 includes a wider range of linguistic categories corresponding to emerging morphology and syntax, with a richer selection of items, than KGNZ-2, as it better reflects the child's growing proficiency.

In the section that follows, we will report the overall performance by Basque-speaking children on these versions of the KGNZ. Our analysis will focus on the gestures in KGNZ-1, vocabulary (comprehension and/or production) in all three KGNZs, and morphosyntax in KGNZ-2 and KGNZ-3.

Participants

Over 2600 questionnaires were collected by May 2011, although some of them were not valid (a considerable number of the questionnaires collected had to be excluded from the database for reasons of incompleteness, age below or above those for which the questionnaire was designed, premature birth of the child, or repeated ear infections, among others). The 2221 valid questionnaires were distributed as follows: data from 442 children were collected with the KGNZ-1 (8–15 months), data from 975 children (16–30 months) were obtained using the KGNZ-2, and data from 704 children between 30 and 50 months of age were collected using the KGNZ-3.

Results

Development across age groups

The following data are presented to show a representative picture of the developmental performance of Basque children. We will provide information obtained from the three questionnaires (KGNZ-1, -2 and -3) on gestures, lexical comprehension, lexical production, morphological production and on morphological complexity.

As the aim of this section is to show developmental results obtained with the whole instrument rather than the comparison of specificities of each of the components, in order to offer a unified account of the results, data obtained across age groups using the corresponding questionnaire in each age period have been collapsed into a continuum, with data grouped by age group in the Figures.

Gestures

Figure 4.3 shows that the number of gestures reported by parents from the list provided in the first of the questionnaires, the KGNZ-1, exhibits a linear increase across the three age groups considered, especially between the first (mean 10 gestures) and the second age group (mean 23 gestures), but also a rise of nine items from the second age group to the last age group (32 gestures).

The most frequent gestures during the 8- to 10-month age range are the following: asking to be lifted up, extending the arm towards a desired object, waving goodbye, clapping games, peekaboo/hide and seek games, and pointing towards an object of interest with the arm or finger. Some new gestures appear between 11 months and 1;1 (13 months): extending the arm and hand to take an object, blowing a kiss, extending the arm to show a held object, holding a telephone to the ear, dance movements, rocking a doll, pushing a car or lorry, shaking the head, swinging, opening and passing the pages of a book in imitation of reading, showing pleasure (yum yum) at eating something, brushing hair, attempting to eat with a knife and fork.

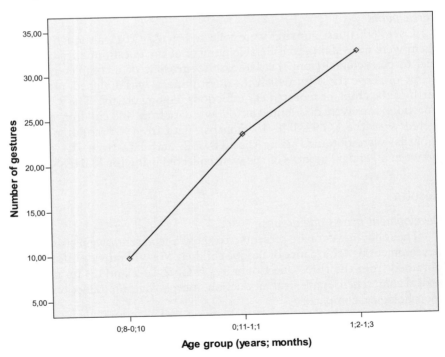

Figure 4.3 Communicative gesture production across age groups according to KGNZ-1

Between age 1;2 and 1;3 they start (acting as if they were) writing, drying their face and hands, nodding or saying 'yes' with the head, using a spoon for mixing liquids, putting on shoes, glasses, necklaces, a watch, and shrugging their shoulders to indicate 'I don't know'.

Lexical comprehension

General comprehension data as measured at the earliest stages of acquisition using the KGNZ-1 questionnaire reveal a linear increase in the comprehension of lexical items with age, as shown in Figure 4.4. As was the case for Figure 4.3, data obtained across different age groups were grouped in three age groups corresponding to three 2–3 month periods. Figure 4.4 shows that KGNZ-1 children between 0;8 and 0;10 comprehend 28 words on average (below 10% of the whole vocabulary list included in the questionnaire), children between 0;11 and 1;1 understand 82 words on average and children 1–3 months older show a comprehensive vocabulary of over 142 words on average. It should be noted that even the latest group (age 1;2–1;3) is far from understanding all the items (below 40%) included in the questionnaire.

The earliest semantic fields reported in the vocabulary inventory before age 0;11 are nouns for people, food, animals and eight verbs, which are *hartu* [take], *begiratu* [look at], *etorri* [come], *erori* [fall], *bota* [throw], *jan* [eat], *eman*

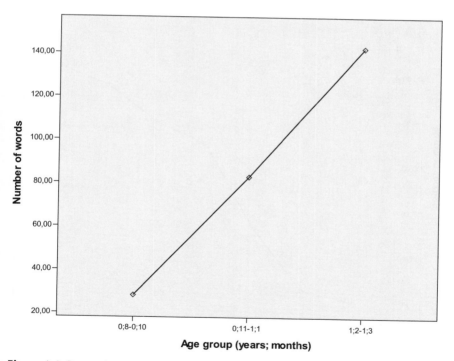

Figure 4.4 Perceptive vocabulary across age groups according to KGNZ-1

[give], *lo egin* [sleep]. The lexical categories reported extend widely around month 12 to vehicles, clothes, toys, small objects in the house and objects outside. Between 1;2 and 1;3 the number of items per semantic field increases considerably, as does the appearance of new semantic fields in children's comprehension inventory, such as furniture, games and routines, adjectives, question words and adverbials.

Lexical production

Figures 4.5–4.7 include production data obtained with the three questionnaires KGNZ-1, -2 and -3 put together and projected on the age continuum represented by seven age groups on the *x*-axis (age in years and months).[2] Figure 4.5 shows productive vocabulary, Figure 4.6 productive morphology and Figure 4.7 productive morphosyntax.

As shown by Barreña and Garcia (2010), word production is almost unattested (with a mean of 2.3 words) during the 0;8–1;0 period and restricted to *aita* [father] and *ama* [mother]. An important increase is observed between 1;6 (mean 26 words at month 18) and one year later (mean 349.3 at 2;6), and again between 3 and 4 years of age (396.8 words at 3;0 and 520.9 at 4;0), although less steeply between 2;8 and 3;4 (Ezeizabarrena *et al.*, 2011).

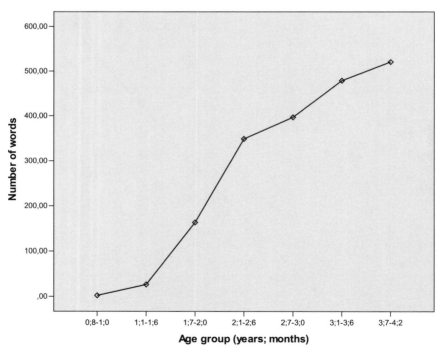

Figure 4.5 Productive vocabulary across age groups according to KGNZ-1, 2 and 3

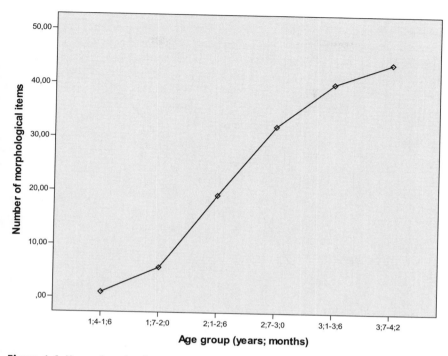

Figure 4.6 Mean of productive morphology across age groups according to KGNZ-2 and 3

Figure 4.5 shows the average number of lexical items produced by the seven age groups.

Proper and common nouns are the most productive word categories in general, and these are almost the exclusive word type during the second year of life, with the exception of some adverbs like *ez* [no] or the verb *jo* [hit], the only verb reported by 2 years of age. A wider variety of semantic categories is reported from age 2 years onwards and before 2;6. Among these, common nouns such as animals, body parts, clothes, small objects and places are found, as well as some personal and demonstrative pronouns, adjectives, verbs and quantifiers. At age 2;6 the list of adverbs, pronouns, question words and connectors increases considerably (Barreña & Garcia, 2010).

Morphology production

The production of (nominal and verbal) inflectional morphology is shown in Figure 4.6. Inflectional morphemes are virtually absent during the first two years. Barreña, Garcia *et al.* (2008) observed that 50% of the children at 1;9 were reported to produce zero suffixes in the nominal domain (number, case and postpositional suffixes) and in the verbal domain, and at age 2 years the same proportion of children were reported to produce a maximum of two grammatical suffixes (case marking) and two or fewer

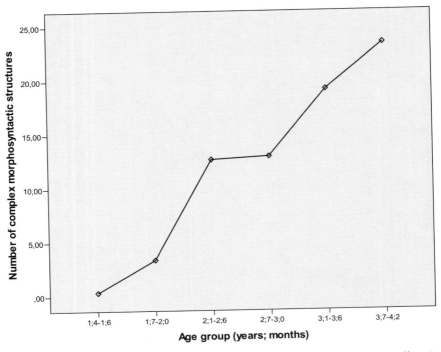

Figure 4.7 Mean of morphosyntactic structures across age groups according to KGNZ-2 and 3

inflected verb forms like *da* [is], *du* [has] or *goazen* [let's go]. Figure 4.6 shows a mean average of morphological markings close to 0 in the period between 1;4 and 1;6 in the nominal domain as well as in the verbal domain. Consequently, the mean production of 5.6 markings by age 1;7–2;0 'announces' the dramatic increase taking place during the next two periods, between 2;1 and 2;6 (mean 19 inflectional markings), and during the next period up to age 3;0 (mean 32 inflectional markings). After age 3;0 the increase slows down, as indicated by the means of 40 and 43 markings observed during the period 3;1–3;6 and 3;7–4;2, respectively. It should be noted that the standard deviation decreases after age 3;0, indicating the stabilization of inter-individual variation at this age.

Morphosyntactic complexity
   The development of morphosyntactic complexity, which can be seen in Figure 4.7, was measured differently from the preceding types of development. Instead of including a list of items that parents should mark, each item in this section included two to three possibilities of answers reported in previous longitudinal corpora. Parents were asked to mark the one(s) their child produced at the time of filling in the questionnaire. Examples in (1) and (2) are items

included in KGNZ-2. Notice that the typology of items included in this section are less homogeneous than in previous sections. Example (1a) shows a kind of error reported in child spontaneous productions in which the placement of negation, participle and auxiliary does not follow the adult pattern (1b).

(1) How does the child say that (s)he does not want something? [item 36 in KGNZ-2]

    (a) Ez   *nahi*   *dut*
        Neg   want   Aux.S1sO3s
        'I don't want/like it'

    (b) Ez   *dut*   *nahi*
        Neg   Aux.S1sO3s   want
        'I don't want/like it'

However, the three possibilities reported in (2) are well-formed verb forms, although the degree of complexity varies from (2a) (root) to (2b) and (2c) (periphrastic forms), as does the degree of adequacy from (2b) (present perfect) to (2c) (past perfect). In this case only the (2c) option can be considered a target answer, indicating that the child is able not only to produce some past inflected forms but to use them in a target-like fashion.

(2) How does your child indicate that somebody came yesterday? (item 23 in KGNZ-2)

    (a) *Etorr-i*
        Come-PF
        'come Participle/to come'

    (b) *Etorr-i*   *da*
        Come-PF   Aux.S3s.Pres
        '(s)he has come/came (today)'

    (c) *Etorr-i*   *zen*
        Come-PF   Aux.S3s.Past
        '(s)he came (before today)'

Figure 4.7 represents the mean values for morphosyntactic complexity obtained with KGNZ-2 and KGNZ-3 after grouping children into six age groups. It should be noted that the first group includes fewer children than the rest of the groups, as it includes children over a shorter (three-month) period of time, namely 1;4 to 1;6, in contrast to the following periods, which span six-month periods or even more. As a general observation, scores are very low (with a mean of about 4, out of a possible score of 37) before age 2;0. A large increase is observed during the first half of the third year of life, from a mean of 4 (before 2;0) to a mean of 14 (2;1–2;6). The increase stabilizes during the next half-year preceding the next almost linear increases to 19 (3;1–3;6) and to 24 in the last age group (3;7–4;2).

Unlike the pattern observed in vocabulary and productive morphology (see Figures 4.5 and 4.6), which are characterized by large increases observed between the ages of 2;0 and 3;6, preceding periods of less intense growth during the last period of the study, the increase in morphosyntactic complexity appears not to start before the age of 2;0, to stop during the next half-year, and to restart again after the age of 3;0, with continual growth up to age 4;2.

The effect of the input on the results of KGNZ questionnaires

As noted, the original intent was to mainly use the KGNZ to measure development in children exposed to Basque from one or both parents from birth, but data from children exposed to varying degrees of bilingual input from parents, grandparents or caretakers were inevitably gathered in the process. Based on information provided by the parents on the amount of exposure to either language, the children were grouped together as Basque monolingual (M) subjects (over 1400); high-input subjects (Bilingual Basque, BB) with exposure of 60–90% Basque (over 400 subjects); approximately balanced input of Basque and Spanish/French (Bilingual Romance, BR), with around 40–60% exposure to Basque (close to 250 subjects); and a low-input group (R, for dominant in Romance [Spanish or French]), with 40% or less Basque input (close to 100 subjects). The sample is not regularly distributed across the four groups, due in part to the fact that the questionnaire was written exclusively in Basque.[3]

In general, most statistically significant differences in development were observed between the groups of children who were exposed to less than 60% Basque, particularly in the later age spans, from approximately 2;2 years of age (Almgren *et al.*, 2007; Barreña *et al.*, 2011a, 2011b; Barreña, Garcia *et al.*, 2008).

Figures 4.8 and 4.9 show the data arranged in relation to the amount of input in Basque and Spanish that the children are reported to have been exposed to. These data have so far only been processed for KGNZ-1 and -2. The effect of input was analysed in several components of the KGNZ.

Production of communicative gestures and lexical comprehension

In the earliest ages recorded in the KGNZ-1 (0;8–1;3), no significant effect of input was observed in the early production of communicative gestures, nor in the comprehension or production of vocabulary ($p > 0.05$) (Barreña, Garcia *et al.*, 2008). The low number of items in gestures and vocabulary below 2 years of age may be the cause of the lack of significant differences across groups M, BB, BR and R.

Lexical production

In general, a very initial state of sporadic production of vocabulary before 1;1 (four words in all groups) is followed by scarce production (mean range across groups 14–30 words, mostly nouns) between 1;1 and 1;6, as shown in Figure 4.8. Production of vocabulary shows a different picture from 1;7

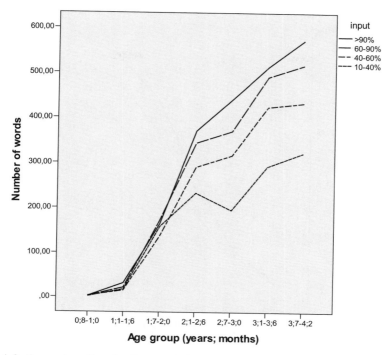

Figure 4.8 Mean rates of productive vocabulary in four input groups across age groups according to KGNZ-1, -2 and -3

onwards (>130 words average in all groups) and especially from 2;1 (mean range 233–371 words). Between-group differences are attested depending on the degree of exposure to the language from age 2 years onwards (see Figure 4.8). From 2;1 to 2;6 onwards, differences between groups reach significant values. The group with the least amount of Basque input (<40%) shows consistently lower values of productive vocabulary than the other groups, whereas bilinguals with balanced exposure to Basque (40–60% or higher, 60–90%) do not always differ before 3;6. The oldest group shows significant differences across the four groups ($p < 0.05$), indicating that differences among input groups become more and more visible as children grow older. In fact, the size of the effect of the input increases from a low at 2;1–2;6 of 5.4% to a high of 20.6% and 30.7% at 2;7–3;0 and 3;7–4;2, respectively.

Morphology production

As with vocabulary production, rates of production of morphological markers increase consistently with age, as do the differences across input groups. Figure 4.9 shows the usage of items out of the total items included in the corresponding questionnaire. Input appears to be insignificant before 2;0, when the mean number of morphemes oscillates between zero and 1.25.

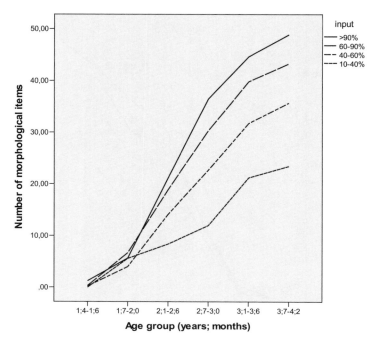

Figure 4.9 Mean rates of productive morphology in four input groups across age groups according to KGNZ-2 and -3

From age 2;0 onwards, all groups produce between four and seven morphemes. The effect of input becomes visible from age 2;6 onwards, although the effect size is low (6%). After age 3;0 the effect size increases considerably, reaching values of 21.4–32.1% between the ages of 3;0 and 4;0 (Barreña *et al.*, 2011b).

Conclusions

The KGNZ or Basque adaptation of the CDI allows the mean numbers of items produced by children acquiring this language to be assessed during their earliest development, between the ages of 0;8 and 4;2. Such items, corresponding to diverse components of language use, such as production of communicative gestures, comprehension and production of vocabulary, and production of morphosyntax, show a gradual increase throughout the period under study, suggesting the suitability of the instrument for assessing linguistic development over a period of time. Moreover, the same instrument allows for the observation of the possible effects of some variables traditionally mentioned as the cause of differences in development, such as biological gender, social class, degree of exposure to the language, and so on.

The last of these, exposure, has been addressed in particular in the final part of this chapter. It can be seen that data collected from children acquiring a minority language such as Basque, where exposure to two languages (Basque and Spanish, or Basque and French) takes place from very early on, reveal differences in lexical and morphological development. Among children with different degrees of exposure to the language, less exposure is related to lower values in the knowledge of productive vocabulary and morphosyntax. The effect of such a variable is barely visible before age 2 years and becomes more apparent after this age (age 2;4 onwards), although with a lower effect prior to age 3 years, and greater differentiation across groups from this age up until the last age period studied.

Similar to other adaptations of the CDI, the Basque version, KGNZ, entailed a language-specific adaptation not only in the vocabulary but also in the grammatical sections. A selection of the items that may better discriminate over age groups seemed to the KGNZ team a basic requirement for the assessment instrument, especially for the KGNZ-3. Moreover, in the case of a postpositional and morphologically rich ergative language like Basque the adaptation has required a specific design for the grammatical section of the instruments KGNZ-1 and -2 and even the addition of a new subsection in KGNZ-3 in order to account for children's early knowledge of grammatical elements like complex verb items, which are very frequent in their input and start to be used productively from 2;4–2;6 onwards. Such structures are an important element in the morphosyntactic development of Basque children and need to be properly measured in order to gain a full assessment of children's grammatical knowledge. Finally, the adaptation into a small and minoritized language like Basque reveals the importance of taking into account factors sometimes disregarded in studies on early multilingual language assessment such as the intensity of the exposure to other linguistic (sub)varieties in contact with the one reported. The convenience of including dialectal variations in the instrument, and of collecting information about the persons using different varieties in their interaction with the child during the earliest stages, allow us to gain a complete picture of children's linguistic performance. That picture includes the influence of some variables such as the input patterns that directly affect children's linguistic performance between the ages covered here, 2–4 years of age.

Acknowledgements

We are extremely grateful to the children, the parents, the caregivers and the teachers who have participated in our research. We would also like to thank our colleagues Nekane Arratibel, Juanjo Zubiri, Alazne Petuña, Amaia Colina, Idoia Olano and Nagore Ipiña for their contribution as members of the research team to multiple aspects of the three questionnaires and the data analysis. This project would not have been possible without them and the financial support of the University of the Basque Country (GIU09-39), the Spanish Ministry of Economy and Competitiveness (FFI2012-37884-C03-01 and -02), the Spanish Ministry of Science and Innovation (FFI2009-13956-C02-01) and the Basque Government (IT676-13). Finally, helpful suggestions and comments by Virginia M. Gathercole led us to improve this text considerably and we extend our heartfelt thanks to her.

Notes

(1) The language features mentioned also distinguish Basque from English, and for that reason they must be taken into account, as they are the main reason for the differences that can be observed in the grammatical part of the original English and the adapted Basque questionnaires.
(2) Numbers corresponding to the 31- to 50-month period (KGNZ-3) have been 'transformed', considering as a reference for such transformation the number of items included in the longest list, the KGNZ-2. Thus, the so-called absolute numbers in such figures are really absolute for the period between 16 and 30 months only. The rest of the numbers, for the 8–15-month period, and the 30–50-month period in Figure 4.5, are numbers extrapolated from the results obtained with a mathematical operation consisting in multiplying the absolute number by the number of items contained in the corresponding section in the KGNZ-2 divided by the number of items of the same section in the corresponding KGNZ-1 (8–15 months) or KGNZ-3 (31–50 months), respectively.
(3) Since in some cases parents did not provide any information about the children's linguistic background on the questionnaires, about 40 subjects from the KGNZ-1 and KGNZ-2 ages were not included and 206 more were excluded from KGNZ-3, leaving a total corpus of 1378 subjects (428 from KGNZ-1 ages and 950 from KGNZ-2 ages up to age 30 months and 704 from 31–50 months).

References

Almgren, M. (2002) La adquisición de la morfología de pasado. No sólo tiempo y aspecto. In *Proceedings of the Second International Bilingualism Symposium/Actas del Segundo Simposio Internacional Bilinguismo* (pp. 183–193). Vigo: Servicio de Publicacións da Universidade de Vigo.
Almgren, M., Ezeizabarrena, M.J. and Garcia, I. (2007) The Basque CDI: Applications in a bilingual society. In M. Ericsson (ed.) *Proceedings from the First European Network Meeting on the Communicative Development Inventories* (pp. 83–92). Gävle, Sweden: Gävle University Press.
Almgren, M. and Idiazabal, I. (2001) Past tense verb forms, discourse context and input features in bilingual and monolingual acquisition of Basque and Spanish. In J. Cenoz and F. Genesee (eds) *Trends in Bilingual Acquisition* (pp. 107–130). Amsterdam/Philadelphia, PA: John Benjamin Publishing.
Arratibel, N., Barreña, A., Pérez-Pereira, M. and Fernández, P. (2005) Comparaciones interlingüísticas euskara-gallego del desarrollo léxico y gramatical infantil. In M.A. Mayor, B. Zubiauz and E. Díez (eds) *Estudios sobre la adquisición del lenguaje* (pp. 983–996). Salamanca: Ediciones Universidad de Salamanca.
Barreña, A. (1995) *Gramatikaren jabekuntza-garapena eta haur euskaldunak [Grammatical Development and Basque Children]*. Bilbao: University of the Basque Country.
Barreña, A., Ezeizabarrena, M.J. and García, I. (2008) Influence of the linguistic environment in the development of lexicon and grammar of Basque bilingual children.

In C. Pérez-Vidal, M. Juan-Garau and A. Bel (eds) *A Portrait of the Young in the New Multilingual Spain* (pp. 86–110). Clevedon: Multilingual Matters.

Barreña, A., Ezeizabarrena, M.J. and García, I. (2011a) La influencia del grado de exposición a una o más lenguas en la adquisición del euskera infantil: léxico y gramática. *Infancia y aprendizaje* 34 (4), 393–408.

Barreña, A., Ezeizabarrena, M.J. and García, I. (2011b) Haur euskaldunen komunikazio garapena neurtzeko KGNZ tresna [The KGNZ, an instrument for measuring Basque children's communicative development]. Paper presented at Euskararen Kontseiluaren VI. garren Jardunaldiak, December 2011, San Sebastian.

Barreña, A. and Garcia, I. (2010) Lehenengo hitzak eta morfologia-markak haur euskaldunengan: elebakarrengan eta elebidunengan [First words and morphological marking of Basque-speaking monolingual and bilingual children]. In I. Idiazabal and A. Barreña (eds) *Ikasteredu elebidunak eta euskararen azterketan (iker)molde berriak. Euskera* 54 (2–1), 603–638. Bilbao: Euskaltzaindia.

Barreña, A., Garcia, I., Ezeizabarrena, M.J., Almgren, M., Arratibel, N., Olano, I. and Barnes, J. (2008) *MacArthur–Bates Komunikazio Garapena Neurtzeko Zerrenda euskarara egokituta. Erabiltzaileentzako Gida eta Eskuliburu teknikoa (Basque adaptation of the MacArthur–Bates Communicative Developmental Inventories)*. Bilbao: Udako Euskal Unibertsitatea.

Basque Institute of Statistics (2004) *Population and Housing Census.* http://en.eustat.es/estadisticas/opt_0/tipo_2/id_97/ti_Euskera/arbol.html#axzz1wUH8IgcY.

Elosegi, K. (1998) *Kasu eta preposizioen jabekuntza-garapena haur elebidun batengan [Case and Prepositions in the Linguistic Development of a Bilingual Child]*. Bilbao: Universidad del País Vasco.

Eusko Jaurlaritza (2006) *IV Encuesta Sociolingüística. Dirección de Política Lingüística.* Bilbao: Eusko Jaurlaritza-Gobierno Vasco.

Eusko Jaurlaritza (2009) *IV Mapa Sociolingüístico. Dirección de Política Lingüística.* Bilbao: Eusko Jaurlaritza-Gobierno Vasco.

Eustat (2011) Alumnado de enseñanza de régimen general de la Comunidad Autonoma de Euskadi 2011–2012, accessed 29 November 2011. http://www.eustat.es.

Ezeizabarrena, M.J. (1996) *Adquisición de la morfología verbal en euskera y castellano por niños bilingües.* Doctoral dissertation, Universidad del País Vasco, Bilbao.

Ezeizabarrena, M.J. (2003) Null subjects and optional infinitives in Basque. In N. Müller (ed.) *(In)vulnerable Domains in Multilingualism* (pp. 83–106). Amsterdam: John Benjamin Publishing.

Ezeizabarrena, M.J., Garcia, I., Almgren, M. and Barreña, A. (2011) A CDI-III for Euskera-speaking children between 30 and 50 months. Paper presented at the 12th Congress of the International Association for the Study of Child Language. 19–23 July 2011, Montreal.

Fenson, L., Dale, P., Reznick J.S., Thal, D., Bates, E., Hartung, J.P., Pethick, S. and Reilly, J. (1993) *MacArthur Communicative Development Inventories: User's Guide and Technical Manual.* Baltimore, MD: Brookes Publishing. [Original copyright assigned 1992.]

Fenson, L., Dale, P.S., Reznick, J.S., Thal, D., Bates, E., Hartung, J.P., Pethick, S. and Reilly, J.S. (2007) *The MacArthur Communicative Development Inventories: User's Guide and Technical Manual* (2nd revised edn). Baltimore: Paul H. Brookes Publishing Co.

García, I., Ezeizabarrena, M.J., Almgren, M. and Errarte, I. (2005) El desarrollo léxico infantil en euskera: una nueva adaptación del test MacArthur. In C. Mayor, B. Zubiauz and E. Díez-Villoria (eds) *Estudios sobre la adquisición del lenguaje. IV Congreso Internacional sobre la Adquisición de las Lenguas del Estado* (pp. 955–966). Salamanca: Universidad de Salamanca.

ISEI-IVEI Eusko Jaurlaritza (2010) The Basque Education System: overview. http://www.isei-ivei.net.

Jackson-Maldonado, D. (2011) A CDI-III for Spanish-speaking children between 30 and 47 months of age. Paper presented at the 12th Congress of the International Association for the Study of Child Language. 19–23 July 2011, Montreal.

Jackson-Maldonado, D., Thal, D., Fenson, L., Marchmann, V., Newton, T. and Conboy, B. (2003) *MacArthur Inventarios del Desarrollo de Habilidades Comunicativas. User's Guide and Technical Manual*. Baltimore: Brookes Publishing.

López-Ornat, S., Gallego, C., Gallo, P., Karousou, A., Mariscal, S. and Martinez, M. (2005) *MacArthur. Inventario de Desarrollo Comunicativo MacArthur*. Madrid: Tesa.

Zubiri, J.J. (1997) *Izen sintagmaren, determinazioaren eta kasuen jabekuntza eta garapena hiru urte arte [The acquisition of noun phrases, determiners and case up to age three]*. Doctoral dissertation, Universidad del País Vasco, Vitoria-Gasteiz.

5 Using Parent Report to Assess Bilingual Vocabulary Acquisition: A Model from Irish

Ciara O'Toole

This chapter describes the adaptation of a parent report instrument on early language development to a bilingual context. Beginning with general issues of adapting tests to any language, particular attention is placed on the issue of using parents as evaluators of child language acquisition of a minority language in a bilingual context. In Ireland, Irish is the first official language and is spoken by about 65,000 people on a daily basis. However, all Irish speakers are bilingual, and children are exposed to the dominant English language at an early age. Using an adaptation of a parent report instrument, 21 typically developing children between 16 and 40 months of age were assessed repeatedly over two years to monitor their language development. The form allowed parents to document their children's vocabulary development in both languages. Results showed that, when knowledge of both languages was accounted for, the children acquired vocabulary at rates similar to those of monolingual speakers and used translational equivalents relatively early in language development. The study also showed that parents of bilingual children could accurately identify and differentiate language development in both of the child's languages. Recommendations for adapting and using parent report instruments in bilingual language acquisition contexts are outlined.

Introduction

Crosslinguistic studies of monolingual language acquisition have demonstrated that for many languages children start babbling from about

6 months of age, show comprehension around 9 months and move to 'first words' (especially for people and objects) at around 12 months (Slobin, 2002). Between 18 and 24 months children move to a period of two-word combinations, albeit with limited morphosyntactic marking, and by 3 years most children have mastered the basic morphological and syntactic structures of the input language (Bornstein & Haynes, 1998). These milestones mean that children who fail to reach them at appropriate ages can be identified early on as having a potential language delay and appropriate intervention can be provided. However, the majority of the world's children are acquiring more than one language in the early years, and the timing and nature of language acquisition in these situations is largely unknown. Furthermore, large variations in language exposure and individual differences in the rate of language development both across and within different languages (Dale & Goodman, 2005) mean that, when bilingual children are assessed in only one of their languages, they are both under- and over-identified as having a language delay (RCSLT, 2006). Without studies involving a representative number of typically developing bilingual and multilingual children, little progress can be made towards the accurate identification of children requiring intervention.

The guidelines for best practice for speech language therapists (SLTs) as outlined by the Royal College of Speech and Language Therapists (RCSLT, 2006) state that assessment of communication skills should take place in all the languages to which that person is exposed. This is because bilingual children can have a smaller vocabulary in one of their languages when compared with monolingual peers, which can be misinterpreted as language impairment (Thordardottir et al., 2006). Thus it is crucial to establish descriptive bilingual norms through appropriate assessment tools. With such tools, a smaller vocabulary size in bilinguals will not be misinterpreted as being below the norm and at the same time the possibility of language impairment will not be rejected simply by the assumption that bilingual children are expected to have smaller vocabularies than their monolingual peers.

Minority language acquisition: The Irish situation

The bilingual situation in the Republic of Ireland is no different from that of other countries, even though Irish, a minority language, is recognized as the first official language of the country. This means that there are statutory language rights for Irish speakers, particularly in the form of the Official Languages Act (Department of Community Rural and Gaeltacht Affairs, 2003), which dictates that all public services, including health and education, must be available in Irish and/or English. Irish is predominantly spoken as a daily community language in officially recognized geographical areas known as the 'Gaeltacht', which are mainly in the provinces of Munster, Connacht and County Donegal, which correspond to the three main dialects of Irish. The population of these areas is estimated to be 96,000 with 68.5% claiming to be Irish speakers (CSO, 2011). In more recent times, Irish has become a growing community language in urban areas of Dublin and Belfast. Moreover, there has been a growth in immersion education through Irish-medium schools known as 'Gaelscoileanna', where approximately 35,000 pupils are receiving their education and engaging in extra-curricular activities through Irish. All of these factors mean that health and education services are coming under pressure to provide for this population, and this includes the ability to profile and measure their language progress. The complication for Irish-speaking children is that they have language skills distributed across two languages (De Houwer, 1995), as all Irish speakers are bilingual, and children are exposed to the majority English language from an early age from a variety of sources. There are currently few resources available to teachers, psychologists and SLTs working with bilingual Irish–English speakers. Brennan (2004) outlines how professionals often translate existing English tests into Irish, although she acknowledges the many pitfalls associated with this practice, not least due to the fact that vast differences between the languages mean that the levels of linguistic difficulty and order of acquisition will not be the same (Pert & Letts, 2001). Assessments developed for monolingual children are clearly inappropriate for bilingual speakers (Gathercole, 2010; Gathercole & Thomas, 2009; Gutiérrez-Clellen, 1996) and so 'a crucial step in advancing and developing services to Irish speakers to approximate the services provided to their English-speaking peers is the development of appropriate assessment tools and relevant developmental normative data' (Brennan, 2004: 34).

Parent report instruments

Dale (1991) discusses the urgent need for valid, cost-effective language assessments at an early age because of the known long-term academic and social consequences of delayed language. A randomized control trial of screening methods in The Netherlands revealed that screening toddlers who present with language delay during a preschool check-up can reduce the percentage of children who attend special school at 8 years by 30% (van Agt et al., 2007). However, young children are notoriously difficult to assess. Some of the key methods used to date include parental diaries, direct assessments and spontaneous language sampling. While language sampling can be useful at the initial stages of collecting normative data for a particular language, and have been useful for investigating language choice, code-switching and the use of morphosyntax in bilinguals, they are not as good at describing children's lexical knowledge (De Houwer, 2009). Furthermore, language sampling has the added disadvantage of being extremely time consuming and restrictive in terms of the linguistic structures observed, while direct testing has performance and situational limitations for children under 3 years (Bornstein & Haynes, 1998). On the other hand, tests that involve parents as reporters of their children's language development provide a far more representative picture of a child's language under 3 years, as parents are more familiar with their child's language development from a wider range of situations (Dale, 1991; Dale *et al.*, 1989). Moreover, as parent report forms can be filled in online or obtained through the post, they enable the collection of rich data from relatively large populations in a cost-effective manner. Among the most widely used parent report instruments are the MacArthur–Bates CDIs (Fenson *et al.*, 2007), and numerous studies have shown them to be effective and efficient tools for assessing early language development, providing a rapid overall evaluation which can serve both screening and research purposes.

The CDIs have now been adapted into over 40 languages, and studies have demonstrated that the vocabulary checklists correlate significantly and positively with laboratory measures of free speech, and non-word repetition (Stokes & Klee, 2009), while grammatical measures correlate with direct measures of morphosyntax including measures of mean length of utterance (Dale, 1991). Their wide-ranging application means that they are slowly coming to the fore in the study of language acquisition in young children. The instruments have been used to explore important theoretical issues, such as estimating the relative contributions of genetic versus environmental factors to the rate of language development (Dionne *et al.*, 2003; Price *et al.*, 2000), and determining the prevalence and predictors of language delay (Horwitz *et al.*, 2003). There are currently three versions of the American-English CDI: the *Words and gestures* scale, which assesses prelinguistic communication and receptive/expressive vocabulary in 8- to 16-month-old children; the *Words and sentences* scale for 16- to 30-month-old children, which looks at expressive vocabulary and early morphosyntax; and the CDI-III for 30- to 37-month-old children, which addresses expressive vocabulary, morphosyntactic and semantic-pragmatic development (Fenson *et al.*, 2007).

Parent report of bilingual language acquisition

Parent report measures have also been used in previous studies of bilingual children. For example, Pearson *et al.* (1993) used the Spanish and English versions of the CDI to compare the language development of bilingual children with monolingual children. For the bilingual children, the two monolingual versions of the CDI were used, and the authors then attempted to disentangle the most appropriate way of interpreting the vocabulary scores derived for the bilingual children in order to compare their scores to monolingual children. As well as the single language measures (for English- and Spanish-only vocabulary) a 'Total Vocabulary' (TV) score was calculated. This was comprised of the total number of words or sound-meaning pairings reported by the parents across the two languages. The authors then mapped between the two versions of the CDI and calculated a 'Total Conceptual Vocabulary' (TCV) score based on the number of concepts that were lexicalized by the children in either language, only counting translational equivalents once. The authors concluded that when TCV was used as a comparative measure, bilingual children had a similar vocabulary size to monolinguals. Junker and Stockman (2002) carried out similar studies using the German and English versions of the CDI with bilingual children, and found that the children had similar vocabulary scores, even if they were only credited for their stronger language. They recommended taking four vocabulary scores from CDIs, including total vocabulary in Language A and Language B as well as the aforementioned TV and TCV.

Although TCV is a more conservative measure of vocabulary knowledge, Pearson *et al.* (1993) caution that it may be misleading in that apparent translational equivalent pairs may not be used in the same way for children as they are for adults. They describe a situation in which a bilingual child used the Spanish word *barco* for sailboats but the English term *boat* for all other kinds of boats. In this case, TCV would actually underestimate a child's vocabulary knowledge as both words would only be counted once. In fact, Thordardottir *et al.* (2006), using the French and English versions of the CDI with monolingual and bilingual children, found that balanced bilingual children (with 50:50 exposure to both languages) scored lower than monolinguals when TCV was used as a comparison, although they had higher vocabulary scores than monolinguals when TV was used as a comparison. These authors concluded that TCV was a better vocabulary measure for children with unequal exposure to their languages, as for those children included in the Pearson *et al.* (1993) and the Junker and Stockman (2002) studies, but TV might be more appropriate for those with balanced exposure to the two languages. Total vocabulary also captured the vocabulary development in a group of Spanish–English bilinguals with on average equal input in both languages more reliably than a single vocabulary measure in a study by Hoff *et al.* (2012). Furthermore, Thordardottir *et al.* (2006) noted that the bilingual children were delayed on vocabulary development in English when compared with the monolingual English group but had similar scores in French when compared with the monolingual French children. This was not the case for Dutch–French bilinguals, who reached vocabulary levels similar to those of monolingual norms in both languages (and better measures than TCV) for children exposed to both languages from birth (De Houwer, 2010). Therefore, in addition to the amount of bilingual exposure to a particular language, language-specific factors might result in differences in vocabulary scores, and this should be considered in bilingual studies using the CDIs.

Other studies that have focused on the issue of translational equivalents in bilinguals include Gatt *et al.*'s (2008) study using the Maltese version of the CDI. This CDI contains some English lexical entries due to the high language contact situation in Malta. These authors compared vocabulary scores reported by parents to scores obtained from spontaneous language samples of 12- to 30-month-old children. They noted that, although parents reported that their children used translational equivalents on the CDI, this was not reflected in the language samples. However, loan words were found in both measures. A study by De Houwer *et al.* (2006) with Dutch and French versions of the CDI found that young children comprehended translational equivalents early in language development. Both studies support the notion that bilingual children understand and produce translational equivalents early in language acquisition.

Finally, Marchman and Martínez-Sussmann (2002) and Marchman *et al.* (2004) carried out a series of studies looking at the validity of using the CDIs with bilinguals by having the parents of bilingual Spanish-English children fill out the form in both languages and comparing the results to spontaneous and structured language measures. They found strong correlations between the various language measures on the CDIs and spontaneous and structured language measures, including vocabulary and grammar, although they noted that within-language correlations were moderate to strong whereas cross-language correlations were weaker and non-significant. The results demonstrated that the association between lexical and grammatical learning did not result from a general cognitive ability, but was linked to the vocabulary and grammar within a particular language. They also noted that parents could accurately report on the child's lexical acquisition in each language, even if they were speakers of both languages themselves.

To summarize, most studies have found the CDIs to be a useful way of assessing and investigating bilingual vocabulary acquisition. Nonetheless, apart from the language contact situation accounted for through the inclusion of some English items in the Maltese adaptation (Gatt *et al.*, 2008), previous studies have used CDIs that were developed for monolingual speakers of each language and used the tests independently to measure vocabulary in children before attempting to map between the two adaptations to determine overall vocabulary size. However, being bilingual is not the same as being monolingual in two languages, and most adaptations of the CDI contain idiosyncrasies related to the target culture and language of the adaptation. This means that it is not possible to completely map directly between the two single-language versions. To date, there are no adaptations of the CDIs for bilingual children, and so this study represents the first of its kind in that all of the lexical items are measured in both languages. This is possible in the Irish context, as early contact with a socially dominant English language is the norm, and so a single parent report form incorporating all aspects of bilingual language acquisition for these languages is appropriate. Furthermore, as there are no monolingual Irish-speaking adults, parents can report on their children's language development in both languages. This study therefore provides a test case for adapting a parent report to a bilingual context. First, the initial adaptation of the checklist from the original CDI to Irish will be outlined, and then how it was used to collect longitudinal data on the vocabulary development of 21 children acquiring Irish as a first language from 16 to 40 months will be explored. Following this analysis, a revision of the CDI for assessing Irish bilingual children and bilingual children in general will be proposed.

Study

Method

Irish adaptation

The initial Irish adaptation of the CDI: *Words and sentences* scale (ICDI) was used in this study. While the adaptation has been described elsewhere (O'Toole & Fletcher, 2008), a brief outline of the vocabulary section will be described here. In the original study the vocabulary items were listed in Irish, and two columns were placed alongside the items so parents could select whether their child used the words in Irish, English or in both languages (translational equivalents) by selecting both columns (Bates *et al.*, 1995). A small excerpt from the original is shown in Figure 5.1.

A number of loan words were also included, in line with the adaptation by Gatt *et al.* (2008). Although there is debate as to whether a lexical item is a 'loan word' or a 'code-switch' (Deuchar, 2008), for the purposes of the current study, a 'loan word' was considered to be any English word which has been naturalized into the phonology, morphosyntax and everyday use of Irish, such as *jeep*. In addition, some Irish words are cognates with English, including *bugaí* /bʌgi/*buggy*, *cairdeagan*/kaɹdəgən/*cardigan* and *moncaí* / mʌŋki/ *monkey*. In this initial adaptation, parents could decide whether they felt the child was using the Irish or English word for loan words and cognates, or both, by selecting the appropriate column(s).

3. FEITHICLÍ (Fíor nó bréagáin) (19) VEHICLES (Real or toy)									
	Gaeilge Irish	Béarla English		Gaeilge Irish	Béarla English			Gaeilge Irish	Béarla English
bád	O	O	JCB	O	O	tochaltóir/ bainteoir		O	O
bus	O	O	jeep	O	O	traein		O	O
carr/ gluaisteán/ mótar	O	O	leoraí	O	O	tarracóir		O	O
eitleán	O	O	long	O	O	trucail		O	O
gluaisrothar	O	O	otharcharr	O	O	veain		O	O
héileacaptar	O	O	pram/bugaí	O	O				
inneall dóiteáin	O	O	rothar	O	O				

Figure 5.1 Vocabulary items on the Irish CDI (O'Toole & Fletcher, 2008)

Participants

All of the families were from the Munster region in the South of Ireland and were required to have Irish as a majority language of the home (spoken at least 60% of the time or more) to participate, although most families reported between 90% and 100% Irish use in the home. In order to establish the level of exposure to Irish among the children, parents completed a language background questionnaire at the beginning of the study to provide a comprehensive picture of the English and Irish input for each child. Parents indicated the primary language(s) of the home as well as the language(s) the child was exposed to from people in regular contact with the child. They also estimated the overall proportion of time that the child was exposed to Irish and English. There were 12 girls and 9 boys, and more of the mothers had Irish as a first language than the fathers. All but one of the mothers were the primary carers of the children on a daily basis, and the other child was looked after by an Irish-speaking child-minder on weekdays from 9 am to 3 pm.

Procedure

Two types of data were collected at each visit: an Irish CDI (ICDI) checklist and a spontaneous language sample to establish the validity of the parent report.

(1) *CDI data.* The parents completed a checklist on the children between the ages of 16 and 40 months over a two year period. Repeated checklists were completed at 6-monthly intervals for children up to 40-months in order to collect longitudinal data. This resulted in 49 checklists overall, with one child contributing four checklists, 10 children three checklists, five children two checklists, and five children just one checklist as they were older when they first took part in the study. At each visit, the parents completed the ICDI and were asked to report on spontaneous production of a word rather than elicited repetition or imitation. The child was credited as saying a word even if s/he did not pronounce it accurately (e.g. /wɑdə/ was accepted for *madra* [dog]). Parents were allowed to include dialectal variants not part of the *caighdeán* or standard language (e.g. *tráigh* for *trá* [beach]) or other word alternatives if the child was not using the standard form (e.g. *casóg* for *cóta* [coat]). However, parents were not allowed to include additional concepts that were not on the checklist. Depending on the age of the child and his/her level of expressive language, the checklist took between 20 and 60 minutes to complete.

(2) *Spontaneous language sample.* In addition, a spontaneous language sample involving the parent and child, of approximately 15 minutes, was videotaped at each time point. The same parent who completed the ICDI checklist was involved in the language sample. Parents were provided

with a standard set of toys (a doll's house containing four dolls, a dog and a car), as well as a selection of Irish picture books, in an attempt to reduce variability across the language samples, and were asked to play with the child as he or she would normally do at home.

Data analysis

From the CDI checklists, a number of vocabulary scores were derived: Total Irish vocabulary (total number of words, excluding any words only known in English), Total English vocabulary (total number of words, excluding all the words the child only knew in Irish), Total Conceptual Vocabulary (TCV, the total number of concepts reported in English only, Irish only and translational equivalents), and Total Vocabulary (TV, words known in both English and Irish). From the videotaped conversational samples, the number of English and Irish words was also coded so that they could be compared to the number of English words noted by parents on the ICDI checklist. Computerized Language Analysis (CLAN; MacWhinney, 2003) was then used to calculate a number of linguistic measures from the speech samples. These included the Number of Different Words in Irish (NDW), based on a 100-utterance sample; D (Richards & Malvern, 1997), a measure of lexical diversity that is argued to be independent of sample size; and the total number of English words. These measures were later used to establish the validity of the Irish CDI, full details of which can be found in O'Toole & Fletcher (2010). For this analysis, the data were treated as cross-sectional and the children were grouped into four age groups ('18-, 24-, 30- and 36-month-olds'), as it was not possible to use each monthly age for comparison due to the limited number of observations at certain ages. As previously outlined, this meant that most children contributed more than one data point.

Results

Vocabulary size

Table 5.1 presents the vocabulary scores obtained from the checklists and the spontaneous samples. As can be seen, all vocabulary measures, whether obtained from the CDI or the spontaneous samples, increased with age. For the younger ages, the standard deviations were larger than the means on most language measures for both the CDI and the spontaneous language samples, reflecting the huge variability in language development at this age. This variability was reduced in the older age groups, although there was still a great deal of variability in the vocabulary measures, particularly in the number of English vocabulary items used in the language samples. Overall, however, the number of words the children knew in English or bilingually (i.e. translational equivalents) increased with age, and so by 36 months of age the children knew over one-quarter of their total vocabulary in both Irish and English.

Table 5.1 Mean vocabulary score on the ICDI and spontaneous language samples

| | Age groups (in months) | | | | | | | |
| | '18-month-olds' 16–21 (n = 10) | | '24-month-olds' 22–27 (n = 11) | | '30-month-olds' 28–33 (n = 13) | | '36-month-olds' 34–40 (n = 14) | |
Measure	Mean (S.D.)	Range	Mean (S.D.)	Range	Mean (S.D.)	Range	Mean (S.D.)	Range
ICDI parent report								
Total Conceptual Vocabulary	81.2 (113.1)	3–378	240.3 (157.4)	20–432	440.1 (214)	115–715	634.7 (141.9)	377–824
Total Vocabulary	86.5 (125.4)	3–417	242.73 (159.4)	20–437	511.62 (296.4)	115–1059	769 (336)	377–1260
Irish (only) vocabulary	70 (91)	3–308	219.9 (143.9)	20–426	345.7 (193.3)	108–658	405.4 (244.9)	53–793
English (only) vocabulary	5.9 (10.3)	0–31	16.6 (19.5)	0–53	28.1 (24.5)	0–89	41.7 (44.2)	0–137
Bilingual vocabulary	5.3 (12.6)	0–39	3.64 (5.2)	0–14	66.1 (128.9)	0–392	187.6 (241.2)	0–535
Language sample								
NDW (100)	26.4 (23.2)	3–60	63.1 (25.4)	24–105	98.9 (27.8)	49–143	117.5 (23.6)	89–174
D	10 (11.5)	1–32	35.2 (26.3)	3–86	59.2 (32.7)	16.3–117.5	80.1 (45.5)	36–195
No. of English words (100)	1.6 (2.9)	0–9	7.9 (9.2)	0–32	10.85 (15.29)	0–60	19.79 (24.38)	1–71

Notes: NDW, number of different words; D, lexical diversity.

In order to examine these data closely, we compared the growth in vocabulary development over the age groups, depending on whether TCV or TV was used as a comparison. A paired sample t-test for the entire group revealed that, as expected, there was a significant difference between TCV and TV for the entire group ($t(48) = 3.15, p \leq 0.01$), with the mean values for TV being higher than TCV. Post-hoc analysis revealed that this difference was only significant after 36 months of age, however ($t(14) = 2.75, p < 0.04$), with the mean total conceptual vocabulary score (694) being lower than the mean total vocabulary (796). The values are represented graphically across the different age groups in Figure 5.2.

Validity

In the language exposure interview, the parents estimated the average percentage of time that Irish was used in the home, and it was reported to be very high, at an average of 92.4% Irish input. This was similar to the 94.5% Irish-only words reported on the ICDI and the 92.2% Irish words found in the spontaneous samples. However, Pearson correlations revealed that there was not a significant association between the reported amount of Irish input with either the reported or observed vocabulary measures. On the other hand, a significantly positive association was found between the various vocabulary measures on the ICDI and direct observations of language from spontaneous language measures. The Pearson correlations for the entire validation sample ($n = 49$) are given in Table 5.2. The correlations controlling for age are shown in brackets. Due to the multiple comparisons involved, statistical significance was set at 0.01 to control for a type-1 error. Apart from D, all spontaneous language measures of vocabulary were based on a 100-utterance sample, as they have been found to be affected by sample size

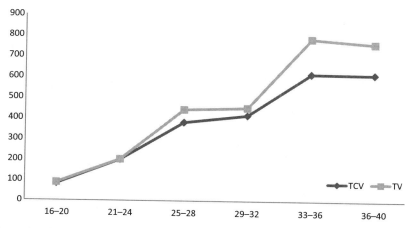

Figure 5.2 Total Vocabulary and Total Conceptual Vocabulary across the ages

Table 5.2 Correlations of vocabulary measures on the ICDI and spontaneous sample

		Spontaneous measure		
		D	NDW (100)	No. English words (100)
ICDI reported measures	Total Conceptual Vocabulary	0.75 (0.56)	0.88 (0.66)	0.50 (0.33*)
	Total Vocabulary	0.71 (0.69)	0.42 (0.39, ns)	0.72 (0.79)
	Total Irish vocabulary	0.71 (0.48)	0.87 (0.64)	0.46 (0.24, ns)
	Total English vocabulary	0.68 (0.59)	0.46 (0.24, ns)	0.83 (0.80)

p values were set at 0.01 to control for type-1 errors; unless otherwise noted, all correlations were significant at p < 0.001.
Notes: *p = .025; df = 46.

(Owen & Leonard, 2002). All correlations including the entire group of children were significant at $p \leq 0.001$. The correlations controlling for age were also significant for the group, except for the relations between the TV and NDW, Total English vocabulary and NDW, and between the Total Irish vocabulary and the number of English words.

Discussion

These results can be reviewed in terms of the validity of a bilingual adaptation of the CDI for capturing children's acquisition of vocabulary. First, when both languages were considered, the vocabulary development of the Irish speakers is in line with that of monolingual children (O'Toole & Fletcher, 2010). For instance, at 24 months, Irish-speaking children knew an average of 240 words (based on TCV); this compares with 292 words for American-English-speaking children (Fenson et al., 2007); 261 for Italian children (Caselli et al., 2001) and 221 for Danish children (Bleses et al., 2008). The vocabulary sizes were also in line with those reported in studies involving other bilingual children (Barrena et al., 2008; Genesee, 2006; Pearson et al., 1993). As outlined in Table 5.2, the children knew 7% of their words in both languages at 18 months, but by 3 years approximately 28% of their total vocabulary consisted of translational equivalents. This is later than in other reported studies of translational equivalents (De Houwer et al., 2006; Gatt et al., 2008) and may be due to the anecdotal reports from parents in this study that they tried to reduce the amount of exposure to English for as long as possible with their young children.

The vocabulary measures derived from the ICDI demonstrated that, in the early years, there was not a large difference between TV and TCV, but after 30 months, as might be expected, TCV was lower than TV. As previously outlined, Patterson and Pearson (2004) and Thordadottir *et al.* (2006) recommend using both TV and TCV measures for bilinguals, and hold that TV should be used for children with equal exposure to both languages so that children with a high proportion of translational equivalents are not misidentified as having small vocabularies. Pearson *et al.* (1993) hold that the most accurate estimate of a bilingual child's true conceptual vocabulary probably lies somewhere between TCV and TV. In the current study, the results indicated that the children were likely to have had dominant exposure to Irish until about 30 months, and then, as their exposure to English increased, they became more balanced. However, as there was a wide range in the number of English-only words used (from 0 to 137 at 36 months), the decision to use TV or TCV as a measure of overall vocabulary size might need to be considered on an individual basis, depending on the language exposure levels of the particular child.

The analysis also considered whether parents' estimates of the amount of exposure to Irish were similar to the number of words in each language reported on the ICDI and observed in the spontaneous language samples. Despite the fact that the estimated percentage of Irish language input was very similar to the overall percentage of Irish words on the ICDI and in spontaneous measures, there was no significant correlation between these measures. This is in contrast to other studies of bilingual language development, including the studies by Patterson (2000) and Pearson *et al.* (1997), who found that parental estimations of the amount of exposure to each language strongly and positively correlated with children's vocabulary growth in each language. In the current study, the lack of association may have been because the language background questions were only completed on the first visit and not on subsequent visits, and because the children were near ceiling on the amount of exposure to Irish estimates and so did not provide sufficient variation to enable correlation. This highlights the importance of regular and repeated language exposure measures when carrying out bilingual language research, not least because the exposure patterns change as the child's language develops, and experiences beyond the home change over time (De Houwer, 2009). It might also have been the case that parents were not accurate in their estimates of language exposure, particularly as Quay (2008) found that parents were not accurate in reporting the amount of exposure to the less dominant language in minority language contexts. This is one of the pitfalls previous researchers have noted in bilingual language research as, despite efforts to gather accurate measurements as to the amount of exposure to each language via interviews and questionnaires, these can be biased by the language choice of the interview (Edwards, 2004).

In contrast to the lack of an observed association between language exposure estimates and reported and observed vocabulary in each language, there was a strong correlation between the number of words the children were reported to say in each language on the ICDI and similar vocabulary measures from the spontaneous language samples. As regards lexical diversity, both D and NDW as derived from the spontaneous samples had strong positive correlations with the measures for Irish and English words reported on the ICDI. In addition, the number of English words reported on the ICDI had the strongest correlation with the number of English words found in the spontaneous sample, indicating that the ICDI captures vocabulary development in both languages well. The data are in line with previous studies using parent report with bilingual children, such as Patterson (2000), who reported strong correlations ($r = 0.91$, $p < 0.01$) between observed and reported measures of language development, and Marchman and Martinez-Sussmann (2002), who found high correlations between the CDI and various spontaneous language measures ($r \geq 0.79$, $p < 0.01$ for all comparisons). This confirms that parents can accurately discriminate children's Irish and English words when completing the Irish CDI, even though they are all speakers of both languages. Marchman and Martinez-Sussmann (2002) reported similar findings for Spanish–English bilingual parents. In the current study, both Total Number of Words (TNW) and D had higher correlations than NDW with the number of English words in the spontaneous language sample. As D is less reliant on sample size than TNW (Richards & Malvern, 1997), it may be a more reliable measure of vocabulary diversity in bilinguals.

Methodological Implications for Using Parent Report with Bilingual Children

This study showed that parental reports can provide an accurate and valid description of bilingual language acquisition in a minority language context. However, Thordardottir et al. (2006) suggest that the ideal procedure for assessing bilingual children would be to develop specific tests that address the unique features of bilingual development, rather than adapting monolingual tests. Therefore, reflection on the results of this study and the CDI format used has led to some revisions to the Irish-English CDI, which will now be outlined. In addition, suggestions for using the CDIs with all bilingual children will be explored.

The first issue was the fact that in the initial adaptation of the CDI to Irish, the words were only listed in Irish and if parents wanted to indicate that their child used the English equivalent, they had to mentally translate the word and then select the 'English' column (as illustrated in Figure 5.1). This was possible in the current study, as all Irish speakers are bilingual; however, it did place an additional demand on the parents. Others reporting in the literature also raised this issue as problematic when using parent report with bilinguals, and so Patterson (2004) recommended using side-by-side translations of vocabulary items. This was in response to a study by Rescorla & Achenback (2002), which stated that bilingual children had delayed vocabulary compared to monolinguals, but which had given parents an English version of the Language Development Survey parent report form (a similar tool to the CDI), but allowed parents to include the Spanish equivalent of a word if their child used that word. Patterson (2004) criticized this method, as parents had to translate the form, placing an additional burden on them. She proposed that using side-by-side translational equivalents of vocabulary items was more valid and reliable for bilingual report forms. In addition, Dale *et al.* (1989) recommended that a recognition format should be used so that parents do not have to rely on memory as they do when vocabulary is presented in only one language. Therefore we developed an updated adaptation of the Irish CDI that lists all vocabulary in Irish and in English to remove this burden on parents, as is illustrated in Figure 5.3. Another issue that arose from the present study was the difficulty parents experienced in determining which language they should decide that cognates and common words belong to (David & Li, 2005; Pearson *et al.*, 1993). For example, the Irish word *traein* /tɟeːn/ and English *train* are pronounced very similarly in Irish and English, even more so when child phonology is considered. As parents are encouraged to credit the child with using a word whether or not they pronounce it accurately on the CDI, it is unlikely that parents can discriminate which language the child is using the word in. There are many words in Irish that are loan words adopted from English and so only subtle phonological differences occur. Furthermore, there are many cognates (e.g. *bus* and *banana* in Irish and English). It is possible that young children are not making a distinction between these word pairs and, at the very least, parents may be unable to determine which language such words belong to. This was also noted as a problem in bilingual situations of typologically close languages such as Galician–Spanish bilinguals (Pérez-Pereira, 2008). Our proposal is to treat such items on the CDI differently from other vocabulary pairs in the child's two languages. Specifically, in the updated adaptation of the Irish CDI, we propose that such words be counted as a single item (as shown in Figure 5.3). For example, while *bád* and *boat* are provided as two options for parents, the cognate *bus* is only listed once, as is the loanword *veain* (*van*). Where alternate

3. *FEITHICLÍ (Fíor nó bréagáin)* (17) VEHICLES (Real or toy)									
bád	O	boat	O	jeep		O	tarracóir	O	tractor	O
bus		O		lorry (leoraí)		O	tochaltóir/ bainteoir	O	digger	O
carr/ mótar/ gluaisteán/ srl.	O	car	O	long	O	ship	O	train (traein)		O	
eitleán	O	airplane	O	otharcharr	O	ambulance	O	truck (trucail)		O	
gluaisrothar	O	motorbike	O	pram/ buggy (bugaí)		O	van (veain)		O	
helicopter (héileacaptar)		O	rothar	O	bike	O			

Figure 5.3 Updated vocabulary checklist

spelling for the Irish words exists, these are included in parentheses, but parents no longer have to decide which language the child uses the item in. This allows for such items to be counted differently from the items for which the two languages differ and they are considered as 'translational equivalents' and so contribute to the TCV score, but not the Irish- or English-only vocabulary score. The benefit of this change is that, in addition to capturing a more accurate depiction of the child's knowledge at any given moment, removing the difficulty of deciding how to treat such words for parents should also make completion of the ICDI faster, as they do not have to reflect on which language their child is using the word in.

The revised version of the Irish CDI includes other aspects that are not relevant to the present study, but which are worthy of mention. First, as a parent report should capture all that is relevant for and unique to bilingual language acquisition, questions regarding code-switching have been included. In the 'grammar' section of the CDI, parents are now invited to provide examples of the type of sentences in which their children code-switch, and the three most recent longest sentences they are asked to provide can now be in either or both (mixed) languages. Secondly, as future research using the test aims to capture bilingual language acquisition for Irish children with varying degrees of bilingualism, the form has been re-adapted so that all of the instructions are in both languages. It is hoped that this will result in more accurate reflection of language exposure and use, and inhibit parents from going into 'monolingual mode', which can be a pitfall of bilingual research (Grosjean, 2004). The ICDI is currently being used with a wider group of children with varying degrees of bilingual language input. It is acknowledged that including a heterogeneous group of children who vary in the amount and consistency of exposure to the languages makes it problematic when trying to identify normative patterns that apply to all children (Genesee, 2006). For this reason, future norms will adapt a model recommended for Welsh vocabulary scores by Gathercole et al. (2008), whereby vocabulary norms are not only related to the child's age, but also to exposure to the language in question. As they have proposed, two types of normative scores will be provided: a general score comparing a given child to all children of the same age, and a second score that indicates a child's placement relative to children with similar language exposure profiles. The intention is that normative information will be available for children from predominantly Irish-only, Irish-English and English-only homes (where children are only exposed to Irish at preschool), as in the Welsh model. As noted in the discussion, however, language exposure information must be obtained through detailed questioning of the parents and should be measured at 6-monthly intervals in longitudinal studies, as it can change over time. It is worth mentioning that, for children who are described as dominant in one language, it may be appropriate to compare their scores to monolingual norms where available, as some studies have found no difference between these measures (Barrena et al., 2008).

For other researchers considering using parent report instruments with young bilingual children, a number of additional considerations are now provided. In the current study, all Irish speakers are also proficient speakers of English and so could report on a child's development in both languages. However, this would be unusual in many other bilingual contexts, and so multiple reporters may be required to complete the form, particularly as many parents will only speak one of the child's languages or some children will learn one language at home, but another in daycare, meaning that neither parent may have sufficient knowledge of the second language to be able to complete both forms. A study by De Houwer *et al.* (2006) had up to three people (e.g. both parents and a regular caretaker) fill out the CDI for Dutch–French bilingual children. They then used a cumulative score to calculate the child's total vocabulary, which credited the child with the best score for any item on the CDI as checked by a single reporter. Therefore, a word was credited as 'understood' if at least one rater indicated that the child understood it in one or either language. De Houwer *et al.* (2006) hold that having multiple reporters may ultimately increase the reliability and inter-individual comparisons of the CDI, and lead to more accurate insight into the structure and nature of early vocabulary in bilinguals. Marchman and Martinez-Sussmann (2002) also found that multiple reporters could provide a view of lexical and grammatical development that was as good as, and sometimes better than, a single reporter. Future studies should therefore consider having a second parent and/or caregiver complete the form, to provide a more representative profile of the child's language skills.

Final Note: Speech Language Therapists Working with Irish Speakers

A recent study in Ireland (O'Toole & Hickey, 2013) interviewed eight SLTs and four psychologists who were employed to provide services to Irish-speaking populations. Preliminary analysis of the themes identified in the interviews highlighted that, although there were significant regional variations in local demand for services in Irish, it was clear that a monolingual model of service delivery was being applied. Therefore, families opted to have their speech and language therapy in either English or Irish, often indicating this on the referral form prior to the appointment. In a bilingual language community where speakers need to have a command of both languages depending on the situation (home, school, peers, wider community, etc.), applying a monolingual model does not meet their needs and may result in parents opting for therapy and additional education services in one language (generally the majority language) rather than in both, and ultimately dropping the minority language.

Another issue that arose was that in Ireland the Department of Education allows for the provision of three hours per week of individual resource teaching for children identified as having specific language impairment (SLI; DES, 2007). However, in order to receive a diagnosis of SLI, children have to have a non-verbal IQ of 90 or more, and have to have received a total language score that is more than two standard deviations below the mean on a standardized language assessment. Often this means that therapists have translated tests in order to test children's language in Irish, and then converted the raw scores achieved into standard scores based on the English norming data. This means that not only is an entirely different population sample being compared for the purpose of establishing a norm-referenced score, but an entirely different language is used. Beyond these issues, there are no psychological assessments available in Irish, and so children are only assessed through English, which may be their weaker language. The professionals expressed their frustration at this, but stated that they had no choice but to continue with this practice so that the children could receive the resources they were entitled to. This practice reflects the reality of current service provision for bilingual populations and the major need to develop appropriate assessments. It is our hope that by helping to develop bilingually normed assessment measures, therapists will be able to capture the language development of these children in both of their languages so those with genuine needs can be identified and receive appropriate intervention.

Conclusions

There may never be large enough numbers of children speaking Irish as their first language available to provide the psychometric properties necessary to provide true 'norms' for tests like those we are developing; the wide variability across dialects, as well as the bilingual status of all Irish speakers, provide further complications. Nonetheless, a descriptive framework for the typical developmental profiles as is provided in the current study is valuable to qualitatively evaluate and compare the language skills of a child suspected of having difficulties (Brennan, 2004). The Irish CDI reliably and conveniently captures children's acquisition of both Irish and English across ages and shows that parents can accurately and reliably report on their child's knowledge of both languages in a single form. It represents the first language assessment of its kind for the Irish language and for addressing the bilingual nature of Irish acquisition, developed to help diagnose and treat those with language delay. It can hopefully lead to the development of more assessments, both for Irish and for other languages. However, further research incorporating revisions to the form to make allowances for the bilingual nature of Irish language acquisition and involving larger groups of children from a variety of language backgrounds is necessary.

Finally, it is interesting to note that the language development of first-language Irish speakers is often neglected when compared to those who learn it as a second language. For example Hickey (2002) noted that in 'naíonraí' (Irish-speaking preschools), children from Irish-only homes only speak Irish in about 50% of their utterances, and so she recommends that specific language plans, syllabi and methodology be in place in these pre-schools to continue to foster these children's knowledge of Irish. She holds that young native speakers of a minority language need the kind of language enrichment that is thought necessary for majority language children from disadvantaged homes. Otherwise, she warns that children will have incomplete competence in their mother tongue, particularly as they are vulnerable to the influence and social status of English, which reaches them through television, the cinema and the community (Baker & Jones, 1998, as cited in Hickey, 2002; see Gathercole & Thomas, 2009). Having an assessment such as the ICDI can be used as a tool (1) to monitor the language acquisition of Irish speakers, (2) to guide the language plans that are needed to ensure that language attrition does not occur, and (3) to ensure that equitable services are provided to bilingual children. As professionals working with bilingual populations have a role to play in maintaining the cultural integrity of children and their families (Ó Murchú, 2001), the development of appropriate assessments and service delivery models needs to continue to be highlighted.

References

Barreña, A., Ezeizabarrena, M.J. and Garcia, I. (2008) Influence of the linguistic environment on the development of the lexicon and grammar of Basque bilingual children. In C. Pérez-Vidal, M. Juan-Garau and A. Bel (eds) *A Portrait of the Young in the New Multilingual Spain* (pp. 86–110). Clevedon: Multilingual Matters.

Bates, E., Dale, P. and Thal, D. (1995) Individual differences and their implications for theories of language development. In P. Fletcher and B. MacWhinney (eds) *The Handbook of Child Language* (pp. 96–151). London: Blackwell.

Bleses, D., Vach, W., Slott, M., Wehberg, S., Thomsen, P., Madsen, T. and Basboll, H. (2008) Early vocabulary in Danish and other languages: A CDI-based comparison. *Journal of Child Language* 35, 619–650.

Bornstein, M. and Haynes, M. (1998) Vocabulary competence in early childhood: Measurement, latent construct and predictive validity. *Child Development* 69 (3), 654–671.

Brennan, S. (2004) *Na chéad chéimeanna: Luathfhorbairt Gaeilge mar phríomhtheanga: Díriú ar an bhfóineolaíocht.* Baile Átha Cliath: Comhdháil Náisiúnta na Gaeilge/Western Health Board.

Caselli, M.C., Casadio, P. and Bates, E. (2001) Lexical development in English and Italian. In M. Tomasello (ed.) *Language Development: Essential Readings in Developmental Psychology.* London: Blackwell.

Central Statistics Office (2012) *Census 2011 Profile 9 What We Know – Education, skills and the Irish language.* Retrieved 20 April 2013. http://www.cso.ie/en/census/census2011reports/census2011profile9whatweknow-educationskillsandtheirishlanguage/

Dale, P. (1991) The validity of a parent report measures of vocabulary and syntax at 24 months. *Journal of Speech and Hearing Research* 34, 565–571.

Dale, P., Bates, E., Reznick, S. and Morrisset, C. (1989) The validity of a parent report instrument of child language at twenty months. *Journal of Child Language* 16, 239–249.

Dale, P., and Goodman, J.C. (2005) Commonality and individual differences in vocabulary growth. In M. Tomasello and D. Slobin (eds) *Beyond Nature-nurture: Essays in Honour of Elizabeth Bates* (pp. 41–81). Mahway, NJ: Lawrence Erlbaum Associates.

David, A. and Wei, L. (2005) *The Composition of the Bilingual Lexicon*. Paper presented at the 4th International Symposium on Bilingualism, Somerville, MA.

De Houwer, A. (1995) Bilingual language acquisition. In P. Fletcher and B. MacWhinney (eds) *The Handbook of Child Language* (pp. 220–250). Oxford: Blackwell.

De Houwer, A. (2009) *Bilingual First Language Acquisition*. Bristol: Multilingual Matters.

De Houwer, A. (2010) Assessing lexical development in bilingual first language acquisition: What can we learn from monolingual norms? In M. Cruz (ed.) *Multilingual Norms* (pp. 279–322). Frankfurt: Peter Lang.

De Houwer, A., Bornstein, M. and De Coster, S. (2006) Early understanding of two words for the same thing: A CDI study of lexical comprehension in infant bilinguals *International Journal of Bilingualism* 10 (3), 331–347.

Department of Community Rural and Gaeltacht Affairs (2003) *The Official Languages Act*. http://www.ahg.gov.ie/en/Irish/OfficialLanguagesAct2003/

DES (2007) *Criteria for Enrolment in Special Classes for Pupils with Specific Speech and Language Disorder*. Athlone: Department of Education and Science, Special Education Section.

Deuchar, M. (2008) *Evaluating Competing Models of Code-switching*. Paper presented at the Models of Interaction in Bilinguals, 24–26 October, Bangor, Wales

Dionne, G., Dale, P.S., Boivin, M. and Plomin, R. (2003) Genetic evidence for bidirectional effects of early lexical and grammatical development. *Child Development* 74, 394–412.

Edwards, J. (2004) Foundations of bilingualism. In T.K. Bhatia and W.C. Richie (eds) *The Handbook of Bilingualism* (pp. 7–31). Oxford: Blackwell.

Fenson, L., Marchman, V.A., Thal, D.J., Dale, P.S., Reznick, J.S. and Bates, E. (2007) *MacArthur–Bates Communicative Development Inventories (CDIs), User's Guide and Technical Manual* (2nd edn). Baltimore, MD: Brookes Publishing.

Gathercole, V.C.M. (2010) Bilingual children: Language and assessment issues for educators. In C. Wood, K. Littleton and J.K. Staarman (eds) *Handbook of Educational Psychology* (pp. 715–749). London: Elsevier.

Gathercole, V.C.M. and Thomas, E.M. (2009) Bilingual first-language development: Dominant language takeover, threatened minority language take-up. *Bilingualism: Language and Cognition* 12, 213–237.

Gathercole, V.C., Thomas, E. and Hughes, E. (2008) Designing a normed receptive vocabulary test for bilingual populations: A model from Welsh. *Bilingual Education and Bilingualism* 11 (6), 678–720.

Gatt, D., Letts, C. and Klee, T. (2008) Lexical mixing in the early productive vocabularies of Maltese children: Implications for intervention. *Clinical Linguistics and Phonetics* 22 (4–5), 267–274.

Genesee, F. (2006) Bilingual first language acquisition in perspective. In P. McCardle and E. Hoff (eds) *Childhood Bilingualism: Research on Infancy Through School Age* (pp. 45–68). Clevedon: Multilingual Matters.

Grosjean, F. (2004) Studying bilinguals: Methodological and conceptual issues. In T.K. Bhatia and W.C. Richie (eds) *The Handbook of Bilingualism* (pp. 32–63). Oxford: Blackwell.

Gutiérrez-Clellen, V. (1996) Language diversity: Implications for assessment. In K.N. Cole, P.S. Dale and D.J. Thal (eds) *Assessment of Communication and Language* (pp. 29–56). Baltimore, MD: Brookes Publishing.

Hickey, T. (2002) *Language Contact In The Minority Language Immersion Preschool*. Paper presented at the 2nd International Symposium on Bilinguals, Vigo, Spain.

Hoff, E., Core, C., Place, S., Rumiche, R., Senor, M. and Parra, M. (2012) Dual language exposure and early bilingual development. *Journal of Child Language* 39, 1–27.

Horwitz, S.M., Irwin, J.R., Briggs-Gowan, M.J., Bosson-Heena, J.M., Mendoza, J. and Carter, A.S. (2003) Language delay in a community cohort of young children. *Journal of the Amercian Academy of Child and Adolescent Psychiatry* 42, 932–940.

Junker, D.A. and Stockman, I.J. (2002) Expressive vocabulary of German-English bilingual toddlers. *American Journal of Speech-Language Pathology* 11, 381–394.

MacWhinney, B. (2003) *Child Language Analyses (CLAN) (Version 23)*. Mahway, NJ: Lawrence Erlbaum Associates. http://childes.psy.cmu.edu/.

Marchman, V.A. and Martínez-Sussmann, C. (2002) Concurrent validity of caregiver/parent report measures of language for children who are learning both English and Spanish. *Journal of Speech, Language and Hearing Research* 45, 983–997.

Marchman, V.A., Martínez-Sussmann, C. and Dale, P.S. (2004) The language-specific nature of grammatical development: Evidence from bilingual language learners. *Developmental Sciences* 7 (2), 212–224.

Ó Murchú, H. (2001) The needs of Irish-speaking bilinguals. *Journal of Clinical Speech and Language Studies* 11, 40–68.

O'Toole, C. and Fletcher, P. (2008) Developing assessment tools for bilingual and minority language acquisition. *Journal of Clinical Speech and Language Studies* 16, 12–27.

O'Toole, C. and Fletcher, P. (2010) Validity of a parent report for Irish speaking toddlers. *First Language* 30 (3), 199.

O'Toole, C. and Hickey, T. (2013) Diagnosing language impairment in bilinguals: Professional experience and perception. *Child Language Teaching & Therapy* 29 (1), 91–109.

Owen, A. and Leonard, L. (2002) Lexical diversity in the spontaneous speech of children with specific language impairment: Application of D. *Journal of Speech, Language and Hearing Research* 45, 927–937.

Patterson, J.L. (2000) Observed and reported vocabulary and word combinations in bilingual toddlers. *Journal of Speech, Language and Hearing Research* 43, 121–128.

Patterson, J.L. and Pearson, B.Z. (2004) Bilingual lexical development: Influences, contexts, and processes. In B. Goldstein (ed.) *Bilingual Language Development and Disorders in Spanish-English Speakers* (pp. 77–104). Baltimore, MD: Brookes Publishing.

Pearson, B.Z., Fernández, S., Lewedag, V. and Oller, D.K. (1997) Input factors in lexical learning of bilingual infants (ages 10 to 30 months). *Applied Psycholinguistics* 18, 41–58.

Pearson, B.Z., Fernández, S.C. and Oller, D.K. (1993) Lexical development in bilingual infants and toddlers: Comparison to monolingual norms. *Language Learning* 43 (1), 93–120.

Pérez-Pereira, M. (2008) Early Galician–Spanish bilingualism: Contrasts with monolingualism. In C. Pérez-Vidal, M. Juan-Garau and A. Bel (eds) *A Portrait of the Young in the New Multilingual Spain* (pp. 39–62). Clevedon: Multilingual Matters.

Pert, S. and Letts, C. (2001) Developing an expressive language assessment for children in Rochdale with a Pakistani heritage background. *Child Language Teaching and Therapy* 19, 268–289.

Price, T.S., Eley, T.C., Dale , P.S., Stevenson, J., Saudino, K. and Plomin, R. (2000) Genetic and environmental covariation between verbal and nonverbal cognitive development in infancy. *Child Development* 71, 948–959.

Quay, S. (2008) Dinner conversations with a trilingual two-year-old: Language socialization in a multilingual context. *First Language* 28, 5–33.

RCSLT (2006) *Communicating Quality 3*. London: Royal College of Speech and Language Therapists.

Rescorla, L. and Achenback, T.M. (2002) Use of the Language Development Survey (LDS) in a national probability sample of children 18 to 35 months old. *Journal of Speech, Language and Hearing Research* 45, 733–743.

Richards, B.J. and Malvern, D.D. (1997) *Quantifying Lexical Diversity in the Study of Language Development.* The New Bulmershe Papers. Reading: University of Reading.

Slobin, D. (2002) Cross-linguistic comparative approaches to language acquisition. In K. Brown (ed.) *Encyclopaedia of Language and Linguistics* (pp. 299–301). London: Elsevier.

Stokes, S.F. and Klee, T. (2009) Factors that influence vocabulary development in two-year-old children. *Journal of Child Psychology and Psychiatry* 50 (4), 498–505.

Thordardottir, E., Rothenbert, A., Rivard, M. and Naves, R. (2006) Bilingual assessment: Can overall proficiency be estimated from separate measurement of two languages? *Journal of Multilingual Communication Disorders* 4 (1), 1–21.

van Agt, H.M.E., van der Stege, H.A., de Ridder-Sluiter, H., Verhoeven, L.T.W. and de Koning, J.K. (2007) A cluster randomised trail of screening for language delay in toddlers: Effects on school performance and language development at age 8. *Pediatrics* 120, 1317–1325.

6 Development of Bilingual Semantic Norms: Can Two Be One?

Elizabeth D. Peña, Lisa M. Bedore and Christine Fiestas

In this chapter we review the purposes of assessment of bilingual children's language. Using the principles of classical test theory we illustrate the process of item analysis and selection. With items from the semantics subtest of the Bilingual English Spanish Assessment – Middle Elementary, we compare bilingual children with different levels of language exposure by item type and language. We then compare children's total scores in each language by language exposure group. Finally, we compare the classification accuracy of bilingual children with and without language impairment (LI), using a total item score in each language followed by a performance on items by type varied by test language and dominance. When the balanced bilinguals are compared to Spanish-dominant and English-dominant bilinguals in their best language only, differences by exposure are minimized. Finally, there were significant differences for children with and without LI. Classification accuracy improved with the subset of items identified with good item discrimination.

Educators evaluate bilingual children's linguistic knowledge for a variety of purposes. In regular educational settings children's language dominance or proficiency is often assessed to determine academic readiness for English language programming. When children fail to reach the expected level of proficiency based on age or language experiences, testing may be conducted to determine if a child has language impairment (LI). In research, questions may focus on proficiency, LI or crosslinguistic comparisons. Although all of these test purposes draw from the same set of skills, the tests used for these purposes may differ in their construction or normative sample. These differences are necessary to ensure that the tests can be used to reliably inform our decisions about bilingual children. In this chapter we discuss the development of a normative group for making reliable conclusions based on the purpose of testing. Next, we draw from classical test theory to present a framework for developing bilingual measures. Then we examine a dataset of bilingual children's semantic performance on the Bilingual English Spanish Assessment – Middle Elementary (BESA-ME) currently in development. We illustrate the process of item analysis by type and population to illustrate the decision-making process in item selection for different purposes. Through comparison of different subsets of bilingual exposure populations and different item sets, we illustrate ways that these test versions can be used to inform research, educational decisions or clinical questions.

Why Assess Bilingual Children's Oral Language Skills?

In clinical settings, speech language pathologists use standardized tests to determine speech and/or language ability. In the area of child language, the diagnostic question typically focuses on whether the child has LI. Standardized tests are employed in order to make comparisons of a particular child's performance against his or her typically developing peers. If performance is significantly below the normal range (often set at 1 or 1.5 standard deviations below the mean, depending on a number of factors including school district policy and/or empirically derived cutoff points), a diagnosis of impairment in the target area can be made.

In research, goals for the assessment of bilingual children's oral language skills may be somewhat distinct. Consistent with the goal of identification of LI, researchers may want to use assessments to rule out LI or to conduct studies comparing children with and without LI. In addition to these aims, researchers may be interested in knowing children's relative exposure to and proficiency in each language in order to interpret experimental or developmental outcomes. Appropriate interpretation of findings crosslinguistically or across different levels of language exposure depends on accurate measures of oral language ability and proficiency. For the purposes of this chapter we distinguish language 'ability' from language 'proficiency'. We define language ability as the capacity for learning language. Language proficiency is used when we refer to a child's familiarity with as well as use and exposure to a given language, independent of ability. Both ability and language exposure are related to language performance.

For children who have exposure to two languages – whether from birth or from early school age – it is often difficult to reliably interpret language test performance for the above purposes. For example, typical performance in comparison to normal (monolingual) peers can be used to rule *out* LI (Kohnert *et al.*, 2006). However, for children who score below the normal range, a diagnosis of LI may be inappropriate if opportunity for learning has not been sufficient. Tests of language ability that focus on markers of LI may not be appropriate for bilingual children who vary in level of language exposure and proficiency. In research, measures to clearly define a participant group are not always available, and test translations cannot be assumed to have the same psychometric properties as the original test. That is, the same scores in different languages may not correspond to equal ability or proficiency (see also Chapter 3 by Letts, this volume).

Ways to Go About Measuring Abilities and Proficiency

For those wishing to accurately assess language *abilities* of bilingual children, a number of options have been proposed and attempted. These include testing in the home language, testing in the 'dominant' language and bilingual testing – that is, testing in both languages. Measurement of language *proficiency* and dominance testing can be challenging. Proficiency testing usually involves a comparison of one of the bilingual child's languages to a (monolingual) norm or standard. Dominance testing more typically assesses relative proficiency in a bilingual's two languages. Each of these procedures necessitates the careful selection of a comparison or normative group, focus on the specific goal for testing, and the development of appropriate and valid items for inclusion on a measure. We will explore each of these below.

Norms

Defining a normative group for bilingual children is a complicated process in the development of bilingual measures for several reasons. First, normative or comparative groups should be drawn depending on the purpose and goal of a test. For the assessment of bilingual language *ability*, bilingual norms are thought to be most appropriate (Bedore & Peña, 2008; Kohnert, 2010; Peña & Bedore, 2009). However, for the assessment of language *proficiency*, monolingual groups are likely to form the more appropriate comparison (Cziko, 1981).

Second, the development of bilingual norms is further complicated because bilinguals vary in the timing of their exposure to the 'second' language and on the amount of exposure to each language. All children have their initial exposure to at least one language at home, but exposure to the other language may also be at home (simultaneous bilinguals, or 2L1 bilinguals) or in the community (usually sequential bilinguals). In the United States, for example, many children start to acquire the second language

(English) when they have their first contact with schooling at preschool or Kindergarten age. Other children have simultaneous exposure to a home language in addition to English from birth. Immigrant children can have exposure to a second language at any time during childhood or adulthood. In our sample of 1198 Latino children drawn from Texas and Utah (Bohman *et al.*, 2010) approximately half of the bilinguals had exposure to English and Spanish from birth while the other half had their first exposure to English in Kindergarten or preschool.

A third complicating factor in defining normative groups of bilinguals is that the amount of time that children spend in each language varies considerably. Some children will have primary exposure to the home language at home and English exposure at school, while others have exposure to the two languages at home and at school. The types of activities and interactional demands also vary according to the language children are exposed to and where they have that exposure (Peña *et al.*, 2002). Thus, it is not unusual to find children who primarily speak a home language other than English at home but English at school. Bilingual children may express different concepts in each language that are related to two different settings (Bedore *et al.*, 2005; Peña & Stubbe Kester, 2004). These factors make the goal of developing diagnostic procedures for the identification of LI highly complex.

Different Purposes: Different Tests?

The purpose of the assessment drives test content, item development and item selection. These same psychometric principles apply to development of tests for use with bilingual children. That is, if the purpose of testing is to identify LI, the test should be one that is sensitive to LI but insensitive to variability in language performance unrelated to LI (such as language proficiency). Here, the goal would be to develop tests in each language that are psychometrically equivalent (Peña, 2007). On the other hand, if the purpose is to conduct crosslinguistic comparisons, then the items should contain the targets that allow those comparisons. In this case, for example, linguistically equivalent items would be included even if the difficulty levels of these items across languages were different. Difficulty differences in the same crosslinguistic targets are based on many factors, including frequency of occurrence and structural differences in the respective languages. Test norms might well be based on monolingual development and organized according to expected mastery of domains or forms.

In the next sections, we apply classical test theory for the purpose of the development of a series of tests for the two distinct functions of the identification of LI in bilinguals and crosslinguistic research. These are not the only purposes for test development, but these are contrasted here to illustrate how item selection differs given these different goals. In demonstrating test development principles for these two goals, we draw from our database of expressive semantics items used in the development of the BESA-ME (Peña *et al.*, in development). In the next sections we first review test development principles and specific applications for our two purposes relative to the assessment of bilingual children. We then describe how to select sets of items to simulate the test development process. We test the resulting item sets to explore how item difficulty and discrimination vary by language experience and how test results are affected by item selection. We use these illustrative examples to consider ways that norms can be developed for bilinguals.

Items

Applying test development principles to the assessment of bilingual children

Allen and Yen (1979) present five basic steps for planning, developing and evaluating a test. The first step in this process is to plan the test. Typically, this means identifying via a table of elements what sections a test will consist of and what kinds of items each section will include. For semantics testing, our table of elements included mode of testing (expressive and receptive) and item type (e.g. word fluency, word relations and associations). Because we were working with bilingual populations and monolingual Spanish and monolingual English populations, additional dimensions included test language (L_A and L_B). Table 6.1 displays the table of elements that we designed for preliminary item development for the semantics subtest of the BESA-ME.

After planning the test, the next step is to write items for all the sections of the test. This ensures that all the item types are systematically represented. For the development of bilingual tests, crosslinguistic methods of *dual focus* and *decentering* (Erkut *et al.*, 1999; Rogers *et al.*, 2003; Sechrest *et al.*, 1972) can be used to ensure that item sets are linguistically and culturally appropriate for the target languages. Applying *dual focus* means beginning from both languages. Thus, as an additional consideration of the test language, we developed half the items in English and half in Spanish using a dual focus approach (Erkut *et al.*, 1999). These items were then translated from the source language to the other language so that there were linguistically equivalent pairs for all items and half originated in each of the two languages. This dual focus approach helps to ensure that the test content represented in the items is drawn from both of the target languages. After translation, 'decentering' (Sechrest *et al.*, 1972) is a process whereby one examines the items to verify that, for each language and culture involved, the concepts expressed and elicited are appropriate. At this point wording might be changed in one or both languages to better elicit responses. This process may result in linguistic inequivalence but often results in items that are better aligned with language-specific linguistic and cultural norms.

The numbers in each cell in Table 6.1 represent the numbers of items developed for the initial phase of test development. For the BESA-ME

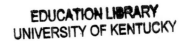

Table 6.1 BESA-ME Semantics Preliminary Test blueprint: linguistically equivalent item set

	Receptive		Expressive		
	Spanish	English	Spanish	English	Example
Categories	8(7)	8(7)	15	15	Rec: Show me all the fish. Exp: Tell me all the animals you can think of.
Functions	8	8	8	8	Rec: Which of these do you use to bake cookies? Exp: What do you do with a spoon?
Characteristic properties	8	8	8(7)	8(7)	Rec: Show me three things that spin. Exp: What shape and color is this present?
Associations	8	8	14	14	Rec: Show me three pictures that go with cooking. Exp: Tell me a word that goes with 'run'.
Definitions	8	8	8	8	Rec: Show me one that is a liquid and dangerous. Exp: Give me a definition of the word 'dentist'.
Similarities & differences	8	8	8(7)	8(7)	Rec: Show me the two invitations that are different from the others. Exp: How are these groups of balloons similar?
Analogies	8	8	8	8	Rec: Show me the best picture to finish this sentence. Dog is to fur as bird is to ____. Exp: Finish this sentence: Leaves are to trees as petals are to _____.
Total	56(55)	56(55)	69(67)	69(67)	

Note: Number of items in parentheses indicates final number of items available for analysis after first round of item tryout.

semantics subtest, we developed an initial 244 items: 112 receptive and 138 expressive. These were further divided by language across seven item types (see Table 6.1). Our target was eight item pairs for each type (defined as Mode x Type x Language). In three cases an item was eliminated from the set when preliminary results indicated that the items could not be reliably scored. Also, for two item types (categories and associations), we had more expressive items to further explore words by level or class. For the purpose of illustration in this chapter, we focus on the 67 items in each language from the resulting expressive item set.

After the items are developed, the tryout set is given to a sample of participants. The size of the participant set can vary dramatically. For bilinguals, larger tryout participant sets are often needed, to examine the role of the language of testing in addition to the characteristics of interest, such as developmental and ability differences. After sufficient numbers of participants are tested, the next step is to conduct a preliminary item analysis. Results from the item analysis are used to reduce the item set for norming. The final steps are then to norm the revised test with a larger, representative group of participants, cross-validate the results and calculate the norms and cut points.

Ultimately, the goal is to select items that are *sensitive* to the trait of interest and *insensitive* to traits that are not of interest. For the purpose of the development of linguistically equivalent tests, it would be important to know which items function similarly across the two languages. On the other hand, to identify LI the goal would be to select items that maximally differentiate children with and without LI but which have minimal discrimination between children with different levels of language proficiency and exposure.

Item analysis using classical test theory

Item analysis is used to examine item difficulty and item discrimination. An advantage of using classical test theory for item analysis is that it can be done with relatively small sample sizes and the calculations are straightforward.

Item difficulty is the percentage (usually expressed in decimal form as a number from 0 to 1) of participants who responded correctly to an item (Friedenberg, 1995). Thus, an item-difficulty level (p-value) of 1.00 means that 100% of the participants got the item right and it is thus very easy; while a p-value of .00 means that none of the participants got the item right and it is extremely difficult. Items at the extreme ends of difficulty – either too difficult or too easy are generally uninformative. These are items that will not discriminate among individuals in a given population.

Item discrimination (D) refers to how well the item discriminates among those who are highly knowledgeable or high performing and those who are less knowledgeable. Applied to the assessment of LI, we examine how individual items discriminate between children who have been identified with LI and those are identified as typically developing (TD) based on a gold standard. Usually the difficulty level for the LI group is subtracted from that of the TD group. Generally, the higher the difference, or the D-value, the more sensitive the item is to the trait of interest. For example, an item that has a p-value of 0.80 for a typical group of children and 0.30 for a group of age-matched children with LI has a D-value of 0.50. Items that have discrimination values of at least 0.3 are considered potentially good items. So, the item in the example would be considered a good item for inclusion on a diagnostic test.

For bilingual children, there is currently no agreed-upon gold standard for identification of LI. In the absence of such a standard, researchers have used several sources of information to make such decisions. These measures include parent and teacher report (Gutiérrez-Clellen & Kreiter, 2003), language sampling (Bedore *et al.*, 2010; Gutiérrez-Clellen *et al.*, 2000; Miller *et al.*, 2006), and clinical judgment (Peña *et al.*, 2007). Applied to the assessment of language ability in bilingual populations, item difficulty and item discrimination analyses should distinguish between children with and without LI against the best available gold standard. Items are selected to maximize differences by ability so that resulting test scores differentiate groups. At the same time, difficulty differences on the basis of language proficiency or language use and exposure should be minimized so that the test does not result in an unacceptable number of false positives or false negatives. Statistically significant differences between children with and without LI are not sufficient. There must also be little to no overlap in the range of performance of the groups in order to maximize classification accuracy.

If parallel tests are being developed (i.e. one for each of two languages), this approach is likely to result in item sets that have different items or item types even if they are psychometrically equivalent. If we are developing a measure for crosslinguistic comparisons, it would be important to have linguistic equivalence – that is, the same number and types of items in each language. However, this may not be satisfactory for the identification of LI because the items are not selected for that purpose. If we want to develop a test that is both psychometrically and linguistically equivalent, an approach to select pairs of items (one for each language) that meet both criteria is needed. Different items are likely to be selected for these two different goals. In the following sections, we illustrate this process of item analysis and selection via the following set of questions:

(1) How does performance on the test for each language vary based on language exposure to the two languages?
(2) How does language exposure affect performance by type of item?
(3) How are test norms and performance affected by item selection, in particular when comparing children with and without LI?

(a) Selection of linguistically equivalent items.

(b) Selection of psychometrically sensitive items.

(4) How can both languages be used in making diagnostic decisions?

Sample Study

Description of the participants

For the purposes of item tryout, a total of 186 Spanish–English bilingual children participated in the study. They ranged in age from 7 years (7;0) to 9 years 11 months (9;11) and had a mean age of 8 years 5 months (8;5). Children were recruited from schools in Central Texas and Boulder, Colorado that served large numbers of Hispanic children. Children were invited to participate in the project if they could complete testing in English and Spanish.

To determine the current use of and exposure to the two languages, we interviewed both the parents and teachers of children who qualified as bilingual. Parents and teachers reported hour by hour what language they (or another interlocutor) used with the child, and the language the child used. For parent information a weekday and weekend day were sampled, and for teachers a school day was sampled. These hour-by-hour reports are combined and weighted to provide an estimate of the percentage of English and Spanish the child uses and hears during a typical week. We report the resulting composites as the percentage of English and Spanish exposure. Classification by exposure rather than test scores allows us to independently examine test performance relative to language experience. All of the children used English and Spanish at least 20% of the time. The children were then divided into three language exposure groups: children who were English-dominant bilinguals had English exposure of at least 60% and Spanish exposure of less than 40%; balanced bilingual children had English and Spanish exposure between 40% and 60%; Spanish-dominant bilingual children had Spanish exposure of 60% or more and up to 40% English exposure.

Children with TD language skills and with LI were recruited to the study. It was necessary to recruit children with LI to ensure that the test items discriminated between the groups of children. Of the total, 37 children had LI as determined by teacher and parent reports of speech and language performance in each language, prior identification by the school-based speech language pathologist and/or a grammatical performance below that expected for their age in the stronger language on narrative samples collected in English and Spanish. To verify that children had LI we required that there be at least three converging concerns out of the four factors available. This process is consistent with best practices for bilingual populations for whom there are no standardized measures available for diagnosis (Bedore & Peña,

Table 6.2 Description of participants

	Spanish-dominant bilinguals		Balanced bilinguals		English-dominant bilinguals	
	TD	LI	TD	LI	TD	LI
N =	55	17	64	13	30	7
Age in months	100.49 (9.67)	96.29 (12.01)	100.48 (10.19)	100.84 (11.74)	103.63 (9.85)	107.00 (9.87)
Percentage English exposure	27%	32%	49%	49%	74%	72%
Percentage Spanish exposure	73%	68%	51%	51%	26%	28%

2008; Kohnert, 2010; Restrepo, 1998). Table 6.2 displays the numbers of children in each group by age, exposure and language ability.

Q1 Language exposure effects on performance in each language

Our first question concerns language experience effects on item difficulty. Logically, children who have greater exposure to one language will have greater facility in that language. At the same time it is unknown how much experience in a given language is necessary before children show equivalent performance on a given task. While it is logical to expect that items that are more challenging for typical children with lower levels of language exposure, it is of interest whether the same kinds of items demonstrate similar degrees of difficulty for children with different levels of bilingual exposure.

For this analysis we first display the average difficulty levels for the children with typical development by language group (Figure 6.1). A repeated-measures ANOVA with test language (Spanish versus English) as the within-subjects variable, and language exposure groups (Spanish-dominant bilingual, balanced bilingual and English-dominant bilingual) as the between-subjects variable was conducted. There were no significant differences by test language or by language exposure groups. However, there was a statistically significant test language by language exposure interaction: $F(2,145) = 35.154, p < 0.001$. Examination of Figure 6.1 illustrates the interaction. Here, we can observe that English-dominant children tended to respond to a larger proportion of English items correctly ($p < 0.05$), while Spanish-dominant bilinguals responded to proportionally more Spanish items correctly ($p < 0.05$). Balanced bilingual children responded correctly to a similar number of items in the two languages.

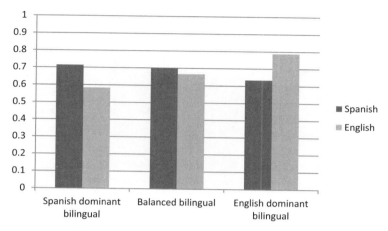

Figure 6.1 Average difficulty by test language and language group

Q2 Language exposure effects on performance by item type

We were also interested in how children with different levels of language exposure performed on different item types. A repeated-measures ANOVA with test language (Spanish versus English) and item type (categorization, functions, characteristic properties, associations, definitions, similarities & differences, and analogies) as the within-subjects variables and language exposure groups (Spanish-dominant bilingual, balanced bilingual and English-dominant bilingual) as the between-subjects variable was conducted. Results indicated a significant main effect by item type, $F(6, 140) = 33.019, p < 0.001$, and no differences by exposure group or test language. There were the following statistically significant interactions: test language by exposure group, $F(2, 145) = 36.608, p < 0.001$; item type by test language, $F(6, 140) = 7.933, p < 0.001$; and test language by exposure group by item type, $F(12, 282) = 2.157, p = 0.014$. Examination of Figure 6.2 illustrates the interactions. Here we can observe that item difficulty for the item type is moderated by different levels of Spanish and English exposure. English-dominant bilinguals performed higher in English than in Spanish on category generation, analogies and functions, ($ps < 0.05$). Balanced bilinguals and English-dominant bilinguals performed higher in English compared to Spanish-dominant bilinguals on category generation and analogies ($ps < 0.05$). English-dominant bilinguals performed better than balanced bilinguals and Spanish-dominant bilinguals on functions and definitions in English ($ps < 0.05$). English-dominant bilinguals scored higher in English than Spanish-dominant bilinguals on associations in English ($p < 0.05$). In Spanish, Spanish-dominant bilinguals and balanced bilinguals performed higher than English-dominant bilinguals on functions in Spanish ($ps < 0.05$).

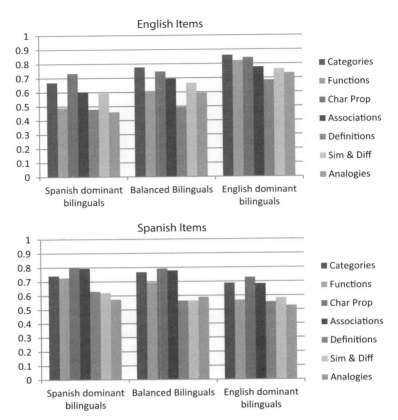

Figure 6.2 Average difficulty by item type and language group

Q3 Comparing children with and without language impairment

We now explore how different levels of language exposure affect patterns of performance between children with and without LI. We consider two solutions for selecting items for inclusion on a test for bilinguals. First, we select items that are translational equivalents to develop linguistically parallel tests. Next, we select items on the basis of item discrimination and difficulty to develop psychometrically parallel tests. For both solutions we compare performance of children with and without LI in each language to illustrate the implications of each method.

Item selection: How are test norms and performance affected by item selection?

Selection of linguistically equivalent items

To address the question of whether linguistically parallel tests differentiate bilingual children with and without LI, we extend the comparison to include children with LI. The scores on these tests represent linguistically equivalent measures because the items comprising them are direct translations. We first conducted a repeated-measures ANOVA with test language as the within-subjects factor and ability (TD versus LI) as the between-subjects factor. There was a significant main effect for ability, $F(1, 183) = 70.788$, $p < 0.001$. There was no statistically significant difference for test language, and no significant interaction. Thus, LI children performed below TD children, but total scores for the Spanish and English versions of the expressive semantics measure were comparable for each group (see Figure 6.3).

Next, discriminant analyses were conducted to examine the classification accuracy of the Spanish and English item sets for TD versus LI children. Results for Spanish yielded a significant canonical correlation of $r = 0.544$, $p < 0.001$. This result indicates a moderate-to-strong correlation between test score and language ability. A cutoff score of 0.566 was empirically derived using the mid-point between the two ability groups' means. This cut score (treating those above it as within TD norms, and those below it as LI) classified 81.2% of the cases accurately with 78.4% sensitivity (correct classification of children with LI) and 81.9% specificity (correct classification of children without LI). Results for English yielded a significant canonical correlation of $r = 0.425$, $p < 0.001$. This result indicates a moderate relation between test score and language ability. As before, the cut score was empirically derived using the mid-point between the two ability group means and fell at 0.548. This cut score classified 72.4% of the cases accurately. Sensitivity was 67.6% and specificity was 73.6%. In this set of results, Spanish total scores yielded more accurate classification than English test scores alone.

In order to improve classification, the measure needs to include only items that are sensitive to ability differences. This procedure is likely to lead to different items and item types across the two languages.

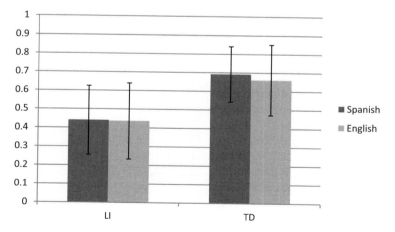

Figure 6.3 Percentage correct: All items by ability and language

Selection of psychometrically sensitive items

The selection of items for psychometrically parallel tests focuses not on linguistic equivalence but on the item statistics of discrimination and difficulty. A primary consideration for selecting items that will be used in a diagnostic test is to select those that are sensitive to the trait being diagnosed, in this case LI. Recall that the greater the difference between the clinical and non-clinical group performance on a given item the greater its sensitivity to the condition of interest, in this case LI. Friedenberg (1995) suggests that items with discrimination values of 0.30 or greater are potential candidates for inclusion on a diagnostic test. We decided to use 0.25 as a cutoff for the first round of item selection. This cutoff point allows for a greater set of items that can be further refined and tested.

In this example, we first determined item difficulty by language group (English-dominant, balanced bilingual, Spanish-dominant) and ability (TD and LI). These data yielded difficulty statistics between 0 and 1. Table 6.3 displays the item statistics for two items drawn from the item set as examples, one in Spanish and one in English. The two items are translation equivalents. We selected items that had item-discrimination values of 0.25 or more for at least two of the three bilingual groups (with no negative values), and at least 0.25 for the three groups averaged. In the example, we can see that for the Spanish version of the item, discrimination is above 0.26 for balanced bilinguals and Spanish-dominant bilinguals. However, English-dominant bilinguals score the same regardless of ability; so, the item is not informative for them. The overall average discrimination is 0.18 for this item. This item would not be retained; the average discrimination for the three groups was too low for this item, likely because the D-score for the English-dominant bilinguals was near 0. In contrast, the English item has discrimination above 0.25 for all three language exposure groups (see Table 6.3), with an average discrimination value of 0.46. This item would be retained. After going through this process, we identified 27 items that met the criteria in each language. The distribution of these items by type is found in Table 6.4. This item set is significantly reduced from the original set of 67–69 expressive

Table 6.3 Item difficulty and discrimination: Translation equivalent items

| | English-dominant bilinguals | | | Balanced bilinguals | | | Spanish-dominant bilinguals | | |
| | Difficulty | | Discrimination | Difficulty | | Discrimination | Difficulty | | Discrimination |
	TD	LI		TD	LI		TD	LI	
Spanish 1	0.70	0.71	−0.01	0.80	0.54	**0.26**	0.95	0.65	**0.30**
English 1	0.93	0.43	**0.50**	0.88	0.46	**0.42**	0.76	0.29	**0.47**

Note: Bolded items indicate those with discrimination values above 0.25.

Table 6.4 Test blueprint: Psychometrically equivalent item set

	Expressive Spanish	Expressive English
Categories	2	3
Functions	2	6
Char Prop	4	4
Associations	6	3
Definitions	3	2
Sim & Diff	6	7
Analogies	4	2
Total	27	27

semantics items. Also note that the distribution of item types is slightly different across languages even though there are the same number of items in each. For categories, characteristic properties, definitions and similarities & differences, similar numbers of items were sensitive to LI in the two languages (across the three levels of language exposure groups). Yet functions and associations had different numbers of items in the two languages that were sensitive to impairment. Specifically, more functions items were sensitive to LI for English, but more associations items were sensitive to impairment in Spanish. Even when there were similar numbers of items for a given item type such as categories, the items that were sensitive to impairment were not necessarily translation equivalents. To illustrate for the items, 'games' and 'shapes' met sensitivity specifications in English, and the items 'limpiar' (clean) and 'figuras' (shapes) met sensitivity specifications in Spanish. This pattern of sensitivity across bilingual children's two languages is consistent with the notion of distributed knowledge (Kohnert & Medina, 2009; Oller *et al.*, 2007; Pearson & Fernández, 1994; Pearson *et al.*, 1995).

Using such a test to discriminate impaired from non-impaired children is informative, but for making direct crosslinguistic comparisons, it is more limited than that of the linguistically parallel example above. Further, the number of items of each type makes it difficult to infer particular crosslinguistic patterns by type of item. While it may be possible to do some crosslinguistic comparisons at the level of the whole test, this solution for the purpose of crosslinguistic analysis is less satisfactory (see Gathercole *et al.*, 2013; Pérez-Tattam *et al.*, 2013).

We examined the mean scores of the children with and without LI on these subsets of 27 sensitive items. As with the linguistically parallel measure, we compared children's scores by ability in each of their languages. We conducted a repeated-measures ANOVA with test language as the within-subjects factor and ability as the between-subjects factor. There was a significant main effect for ability, $F(1, 183) = 129.348$, $p < 0.001$. There was no statistically significant difference for test language, and no significant interaction.

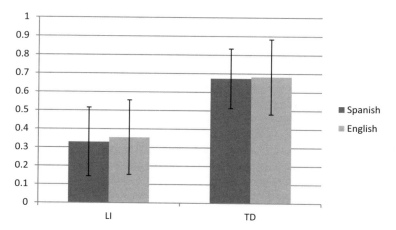

Figure 6.4 Percentage correct: selected most discriminant items by ability and language

Thus, as with the total item set, the total scores for the selected subset of most discriminant items were comparable for the Spanish and English versions of the expressive semantics measure (see Figure 6.4).

Next, discriminant analyses were conducted to examine the classification accuracy of the reduced Spanish and English item sets for TD and LI children. Results for Spanish yielded a significant canonical correlation of $r = 0.641$, $p < 0.001$. This result indicates a strong correlation between test score and language ability. The cut score was 0.501, empirically derived using the mid-point between the two ability groups' means. This cut score classified 85.9% of the cases accurately with 81.1% sensitivity and 87.2% specificity. This classification rate is an improvement over using the version representing the linguistically equivalent item set above. Results for English yielded a significant canonical correlation of $r = 0.546$, $p < 0.001$. This result indicates a moderate-to-strong association between test score and language ability. As before, the cut score was empirically derived using the mid-point between the two ability group means and fell at 0.518. This cut score classified 77.3% of the cases accurately. Sensitivity was 78.4% and specificity was 77.0%. In this set of results, Spanish total scores yielded more accurate classification than English test scores alone. However, the psychometrically parallel versions for both languages demonstrate improved classification rates compared to the linguistically equivalent versions.

Q4 Using both languages to make diagnostic decisions for bilingual children

A well-known challenge in the assessment of language ability in bilingual children is differentiating between those with true LI and those who are typically developing. The last 10 years has seen increased knowledge about the trajectory of typical second language learning and typical bilingualism at different stages of development (Álvarez, 2003; Bedore *et al.*, 2006; Fusté-Herrmann *et al.*, 2006; Gutiérrez-Clellen, 2002; Gutiérrez-Clellen *et al.*, 2000; Sheng *et al.*, 2006). Similarly, in the area of bilingual LI there is emerging databased information that helps clinicians and educators make decisions about LI (Bedore *et al.*, 2010; Gutiérrez-Clellen *et al.*, 2006, 2008; Håkansson *et al.*, 2003; Jacobson & Schwartz, 2005; Kohnert *et al.*, 2006; McCabe & Bliss, 2004; Paradis *et al.*, 2003).

One question for the assessment of bilinguals is how to incorporate information from two languages when making a diagnostic decision. There is general agreement that language testing of bilinguals should consider both languages, and a number of researchers have advocated testing in two languages (Bedore & Peña, 2008; Gutiérrez-Clellen, 1999; Kohnert, 2010). Clinically, we expect that children who have true LI would demonstrate delays in both of their languages. Testing in two languages has been used to confirm or exclude bilingual participants for research using standardized testing (Paradis *et al.*, 2003; Windsor & Kohnert, 2004). In this section, we compare our two test solutions (linguistically equivalent and psychometrically equivalent tests) to further illustrate the challenges and possible solutions to accurately differentiating bilingual children with and without LI. We conducted discriminant analyses for each of the two sets of measures, this time entering both Spanish and English scores into the analysis. We entered both English and Spanish total percentage scores to determine if both languages together improved classification for this group of bilingual children.

Combining two languages using linguistically equivalent measures

We first tested this idea using the linguistically equivalent measures. Results for both languages show a significant canonical correlation with ability of $r = 0.551$, $p < 0.001$, which indicates a moderate-to-strong correlation between test score and language ability. Overall, 80% of the cases were correctly classified. Sensitivity was 75.7% and specificity was 81.1%. These classification results are an improvement over using English total scores alone, but similar to the results for Spanish total scores alone. Figure 6.5 displays the ability group means in an *x-y* scatterplot. The scatterplot allows examination of both languages together. As can be observed, the group means are statistically different, yet there is some overlap, as indicated by the standard deviation error bars. Children who scored in this overlapped area in both languages are those who are most likely to be misclassified. Thus, while the linguistically parallel versions of the measures allow direct comparison by item, item type and level of fluency, they only do a fair job of accurately classifying the children by ability. This pattern of overlap means that it would be very difficult to differentiate accurately among children with and without LI on the basis of the linguistically equivalent measures.

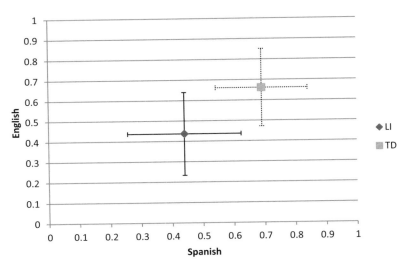

Figure 6.5 *X-Y* plot of Spanish and English means based on all items for children with and without LI

Comparing LI and TD children using psychometrically equivalent measures

The next solution focuses on the psychometrically equivalent tests. As before, we conducted discriminant analyses, entering both Spanish and English scores simultaneously. The function yielded a canonical correlation of $r = 0.657$, $p < 0.001$, which is considered strong. Correct classification overall was with 83.8% sensitivity and specificity at 83.8%. Compared to the classification rate of the linguistically equivalent measures, this classification rate is higher. Compared to the classification rate of the parallel equivalent tasks this rate shows mixed improvement. Compared to Spanish alone, sensitivity is improved, but this is at the cost of reduced specificity. Compared to English alone, both sensitivity and specificity improve.

The improved classification rate is illustrated in Figure 6.6 in an in an *x-y* scatterplot. As can be observed, the group means are statistically different. We also see that there is little overlap in the range of performance between the children with and without LI. Thus, misclassifications are reduced.

Conclusions

The focus of this chapter has been test development for the assessment of bilingual children. There are three key points to keep in mind. First, selection of items depends on the purpose of the test. Related to this first key point, the comparison population used for a given test also depends on what

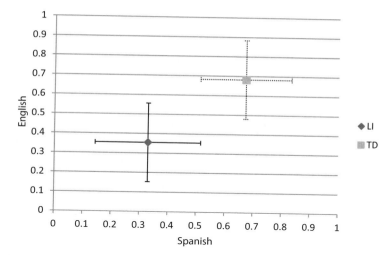

Figure 6.6 *X-Y* plot of Spanish and English means based on selected most discriminant items for children with and without LI

the test will be used for. Second, a focus on linguistic versus psychometrically equivalent tests is likely to show different patterns of performance in bilingual children. Third, when using tests for assessing the language abilities in bilingual children, it is important to test in both languages and use the information simultaneously.

As illustrated in this chapter, children perform differently on semantic items depending on the language of testing and depending on the population. One reason that children may perform differently across languages on items is that the frequency of occurrence of those items is different. These differences may be due to the structure of the languages, cultural differences and environmental differences. An example can be found by comparing frequency data in the *Corpus del Español* (Davies, 2002) and *The Corpus of Contemporary American English* (Davies, 2008). Comparisons by parts of speech indicate comparable frequencies for nouns, adverbs and adjectives in spoken language overall. But the frequency of English pronouns (93,410/ million) is higher than that of Spanish pronouns (73,150/million), while Spanish has a higher frequency of articles (105,910/million) than English (71,476/million). Another source of crosslinguistic difference has to do with cultural and environmental factors. In Peña *et al.* (2002) we found that items generated in Spanish versus English on a category fluency task were often tied to experiences in a given language. For example, in the food category children generated items in Spanish that were associated with family events while those in English were more associated with school and peer-interactions.

For the purpose of making crosslinguistic comparisons it was important to have items or item-types that were represented equally in both languages. For this comparison we were able to examine patterns of performance that were related to level of proficiency/experience in Spanish and English and differences. On the other hand, for the purpose of identification of LI, we saw that the same items did not differentiate among children well. For that purpose we needed instead to select items that were sensitive to impairment, to maximize those differences for the purpose of making an accurate diagnosis.

A central tenet in classical test theory is that norms are dependent on the population. Applied to bilingual norms, it is important to understand the purpose of the test in order to make the proper comparison. For assessment of fluency or mastery in a language it is important to compare with a population that is monolingual because the question focuses on how close students are to native-like proficiency (Cziko, 1981). A slightly different group, however, might be needed when making diagnostic decisions in a bilingual population. Bilingual children, due to their mixed dominance and knowledge in each language, should be compared to other bilingual children. Understanding the effects of different levels of language exposure can help us to better make decisions about LI by controlling for these different bilingual experiences.

Examination of these patterns simultaneously, such as in the x-y graphs presented here, can assist in visualizing and comparing bilingual children's performance in each language and can help to compare differences systematically so that accurate decisions can be made.

References

Allen, M. and Yen, W. (1979) *Introduction to Measurement Theory*. Belmont, CA: Wadsworth.

Álvarez, E. (2003) Character introduction in two languages: Its development in the stories of a Spanish–English bilingual child age 6; 11–10; 11. *Bilingualism: Language and Cognition* 6 (3), 227–243.

Bedore, L.M., Fiestas, C.E., Peña, E.D. and Nagy, V. (2006) Maze use in narratives of bilingual and functionally monolingual children. *Bilingualism: Language and Cognition* 9, 233–247.

Bedore, L.M. and Peña, E.D. (2008) Assessment of bilingual children for identification of language impairment: Current findings and implications for practice. *International Journal of Bilingual Education and Bilingualism* 11 (1), 1–29.

Bedore, L.M., Peña, E.D., García, M. and Cortez, C. (2005) Conceptual versus monolingual scoring: When does it make a difference? *Speech, Language, Hearing Services in Schools* 36, 188–200.

Bedore, L.M., Peña, E.D., Gillam, R.B. and Ho, T.-H. (2010) Language sample measures and language ability in Spanish–English bilingual kindergarteners. *Journal of Communication Disorders* 43 (6), 498–510; doi: 10.1016/j.jcomdis.2010.05.002.

Bohman, T.M., Bedore, L.M., Peña, E.D., Mendez-Perez, A. and Gillam, R.B. (2010) What you hear and what you say: Language performance in Spanish–English bilinguals. *International Journal of Bilingual Education and Bilingualism* 13 (3), 325–344; doi: 10.1080/13670050903342019.

Cziko, G.A. (1981) Psychometric and edumetric approaches to language testing: Implications and applications. *Applied Linguistics* 2, 27–34.

Davies, M. (2002) *Corpus del Español (100 Million Words, 1200s–1900s).* Washington, DC: National Endowment for the Humanities. http://www.corpusdelespanol.org.

Davies, M. (2008) *The Corpus of Contemporary American English (COCA): 385 Million Words, 1990-Present.* Provo, UT: Brigham Young University. http://corpus.byu.edu/coca/.

Erkut, S., Alarcón, O., Coll, C.G., Tropp, L.R. and García, H.A.V. (1999) The dual-focus approach to creating bilingual measures. *Journal of Cross-Cultural Psychology* 30 (2), 206–218.

Friedenberg, L. (1995) *Psychological Testing: Design, Analysis, and Use.* Needham Heights, MA: Allyn and Bacon.

Fusté-Herrmann, B., Silliman, E.R., Bahr, R.H., Fasnacht, K.S. and Federico, J.E. (2006) Mental state verb production in the oral narratives of English- and Spanish-speaking preadolescents: An exploratory study of lexical diversity and depth. *Learning Disabilities Research & Practice* 21 (1), 44–60.

Gathercole, V.C.M., Thomas, E.M., Roberts, E., Hughes, C. and Hughes, E.K. (2013) Why assessment needs to take exposure into account: Vocabulary and grammatical abilities in bilingual children. In V.C.M. Gathercole (ed.) *Issues in the Assessment of Bilinguals* (pp. 20–55). Bristol: Multilingual Matters.

Gutiérrez-Clellen, V.F. (1999) Language choice in intervention with bilingual children. *American Journal of Speech Language Pathology* 8 (4), 291–302.

Gutiérrez-Clellen, V.F. (2002) Narratives in two languages: Assessing performance of bilingual children. *Linguistics and Education* 13 (2), 175–197.

Gutiérrez-Clellen, V.F. and Kreiter, J. (2003) Understanding child bilingual acquisition using parent and teacher reports. *Applied Psycholinguistics* 24 (2), 267–288.

Gutiérrez-Clellen, V.F., Restrepo, M.A., Bedore, L.M., Peña, E.D. and Anderson, R.T. (2000) Language sample analysis in Spanish-speaking children: Methodological considerations. *Language, Speech & Hearing Services in the Schools* 31 (1), 88–98.

Gutiérrez-Clellen, V.F., Restrepo, M.A. and Simon-Cereijido, G. (2006) Evaluating the discriminant accuracy of a grammatical measure with Spanish-speaking children. *Journal of Speech Language & Hearing Research* 49 (6), 1209–1223.

Gutiérrez-Clellen, V.F., Simon-Cereijido, G. and Wagner, C. (2008) Bilingual children with language impairment: A comparison with monolinguals and second language learners. *Applied Psycholinguistics* 29 (1), 3–19.

Håkansson, G., Salameh, E-K. and Nettelbladt, U. (2003) Measuring language development in bilingual children: Swedish-Arabic children with and without language impairment. *Linguistics* 41 (2), 255.

Jacobson, P.F. and Schwartz, R.G. (2005) English past tense use with bilingual children with language impairment. *American Journal of Speech Language Pathology* 14 (4), 313–323.

Kohnert, K. (2010) Bilingual children with primary language impairment: Issues, evidence and implications for clinical actions. *Journal of Communication Disorders* 43 (6), 456–473. doi: 10.1016/j.jcomdis.2010.02.002.

Kohnert, K. and Medina, A. (2009) Bilingual children and communication disorders: A 30-year research retrospective. *Seminars in Speech and Language* 30 (4), 219–233. doi: 10.1055/s-0029-1241721.

Kohnert, K., Windsor, J. and Yim, D. (2006) Do language-based processing tasks separate children with language impairment from typical bilinguals? *Learning Disabilities Research & Practice* 21 (1), 19–29.

McCabe, A. and Bliss, L.S. (2004) Narratives from Spanish-speaking children with impaired and typical language development. *Imagination, Cognition and Personality* 24 (4), 331–346.

Miller, J.F., Heilmann, J., Nockerts, A., Iglesias, A., Fabiano, L. and Francis, D.J. (2006) Oral language and reading in bilingual children. *Learning Disabilities Research & Practice* 21 (1), 30–43.

Oller, D.K., Pearson, B.Z. and Cobo-Lewis, A.B. (2007) Profile effects in early bilingual language and literacy. *Applied Psycholinguistics* 28 (2), 191–230.
Paradis, J., Crago, M., Genesee, F. and Rice, M. (2003) French–English bilingual children with SLI: How do they compare with their monolingual peers? *Journal of Speech Language & Hearing Research* 46 (1), 113.
Pearson, B.Z. and Fernández, S.C. (1994) Patterns of interaction in the lexical growth in two languages of bilingual infants and toddlers. *Language Learning* 44 (4), 617–653.
Pearson, B.Z., Fernández, S.C. and Oller, D.K. (1995) Cross-language synonyms in the lexicons of bilingual infants: One language or two? *Journal of Child Language* 22 (2), 345–368.
Peña, E.D. (2007) Lost in translation: Methodological considerations in cross-cultural research. *Child Development* 78 (4), 1255–1264.
Peña, E.D. and Bedore, L.M. (2009) Bilingualism in child language disorders. In R.G. Schwartz (ed.) *Handbook of Child Language Disorders* (pp. 281–307). New York: Psychology Press.
Peña, E.D., Bedore, L.M., Iglesias, A., Gutiérrez-Clellen, V.F. and Goldstein, B. (in development) *Bilingual English Spanish Assessment – Middle Elementary (BESA-ME)*.
Peña, E.D., Bedore, L.M. and Zlatic-Guinta, R. (2002) Category-generation performance of bilingual children: The influence of condition, category, and language. *Journal of Speech Language & Hearing Research* 45, 938–947.
Peña, E.D., Reséndiz, M. and Gillam, R.B. (2007) The role of clinical judgments of modifiability in the diagnosis of language impairment. *Advances in Speech Language Pathology* 9 (4), 332–345.
Peña, E.D. and Stubbe Kester, E. (2004) Semantic development in Spanish–English bilinguals: Theory, assessment, and intervention. In B. Goldstein (ed.) *Bilingual Language Development and Disorders in Spanish-English Speakers*. Baltimore, MD: Brookes Publishing.
Pérez-Tattam, R., Gathercole, V.C.M., Yavas, F. and Stadthagen-González, H. (2013) Measuring grammatical knowledge and abilities in bilinguals: Implications for assessment and testing. In V.C.M. Gathercole (ed.) *Issues in the Assessment of Bilinguals* (pp. 111–129). Bristol: Multilingual Matters.
Restrepo, M.A. (1998) Identifiers of predominantly Spanish-speaking children with language impairment. *Journal of Speech Language & Hearing Research* 41 (6), 1398–1411.
Rogers, W.T., Gierl, M.J., Tardif, C., Lin, J. and Rinaldi, C. (2003) Differential validity and utility of successive and simultaneous approaches to the development of equivalent achievement tests in French and English. *Alberta Journal of Educational Research* 49 (3), 290–304.
Sechrest, L., Fay, T.L. and Hafeez Zaidi, S.M. (1972) Problems of translation in cross-cultural research. *Journal of Cross-Cultural Psychology* 3 (1), 41–56.
Sheng, L., McGregor, K.K. and Marian, V. (2006) Lexical-semantic organization in bilingual children: Evidence from a repeated word association task. *Journal of Speech, Language, and Hearing Research* 49 (3), 572–587.
Windsor, J. and Kohnert, K. (2004) The search for common ground: Part 1. Lexical performance by linguistically diverse learners. *Journal of Speech and Hearing Research* 47, 877–890.

7 Vocabulary Assessment of Bilingual Adults: To Cognate or Not to Cognate

Hans Stadthagen-González,
Virginia C. Mueller Gathercole,
Rocío Pérez-Tattam and Feryal Yavas

In this chapter we present the results of a study in which adult Spanish–English bilinguals completed two standardized receptive vocabulary measures, the PPVT and the TVIP. Participants also completed an extensive background questionnaire which included items probing their language experience in different domains as they were growing up, as well as socio-economic status and education. Participants' performance relative to one another, according to level of early bilingual exposure, and to monolinguals is reported, as well as both 'external' and 'internal' factors that potentially influence performance. We found that vocabulary scores in Spanish and English were highly correlated for all bilingual groups, and that all bilingual groups performed generally above the norm in both languages. Furthermore, we found evidence of a lasting relationship between the bilinguals' linguistic experience as children and their current performance on Spanish receptive vocabulary, but all bilinguals seem to have 'topped up' in English. We found that bilinguals showed a modest but highly significant advantage for cognates over non-cognates within their vocabulary range, indicating that they make use of some of their Spanish knowledge while completing the English vocabulary test. Furthermore, we introduce the idea of 'intuitive' cognates, that is, English words that can be recognized by Spanish monolinguals, to contrast with linguistic cognates. We found that not all linguistic cognates are recognized as such by Spanish monolinguals. Bilingual participants showed a small but significant advantage in the accuracy rate for intuitive over linguistic cognates. We discuss the implications of these findings for the assessment of vocabulary in bilinguals.

Vocabulary knowledge is central to knowledge of a language. It is the earliest component of the morphosyntactic system to be learned by young children, it sets the foundation for syntactic development and it correlates highly with syntactic abilities at multiple levels (e.g. Bates & Goodman, 1997, 1999; Bates et al., 1994, 1995; Conboy & Thal, 2006; Conti-Ramsden & Jones, 1997; Dale et al., 2000; Fenson et al., 1994; Jones & Conti-Ramsden, 1997). Assessment of vocabulary is at the heart of any language assessment, whether of mono-lingual or bilingual populations, whether of children or adults. Much of the work on the assessment of bilinguals focuses on children in the process of learning two languages and attempts to tease apart the factors that may be ongoing influences in that acquisition. Those factors include the level of exposure to the language in the home, the language mix and dominance rela-tions in the community, usage across contexts, the relationship between the two languages being learned, and socio-economic influences, among others. Many of the chapters in this volume examine such matters in detail. In this chapter, however, we will examine these from the perspective of bilingual adults who have arrived at the end state of the process of learning their two languages. By exploring the long-lasting influence of such factors on the ulti-mate attainment in each of the two languages, we can gain a more compre-hensive understanding of lexical knowledge in bilinguals and, as a result, can better reflect on the optimal assessment of vocabulary abilities in bilinguals at any age.

Our focus here is on adults who grew up as bilinguals in Miami. In all cases, the two languages being learned were Spanish and English and, in all cases, the bilinguals were high-functioning, highly educated individuals, enrolled in or having completed tertiary education in English. We used two readily available and widely used standardized tests of vocabulary in English and Spanish, the PPVT-4 Form A (*Peabody Picture Vocabulary Test*, 4th edn; Dunn & Dunn, 2007) and the TVIP-H (*Test de Vocabulario en Imágenes Peabody Adaptación Hispanoamericana*; Dunn et al., 1986). We report on performance on these two tests, with a focus on several key questions:

(a)   How do bilinguals perform relative to monolinguals?
(b)   What influence have 'external' factors had on bilinguals' ultimate attain-ment? These might include, for example:
    (i)   the type of exposure they had to the two languages in childhood;
    (ii)   who spoke which language to them;
    (iii) which language(s) they spoke to parents, siblings and friends; and
    (iv)   possible socio-economic factors, such as parental educational levels.
(c)   What influence have factors 'internal' to the languages and the bilin-guals' knowledge of two languages had on ultimate lexical knowledge? We examine in particular how lexical knowledge is influenced in bilin-guals by the presence of interlanguage cognates, i.e. words that look/sound similar and mean similar things (e.g. *carro* and *car*).

The answers to these questions have important ramifications for expectations regarding bilinguals' knowledge of their two languages and, hence, for assessment of bilinguals' vocabulary abilities, and for future directions in the development and interpretation of such measures.

Background

It is by now well documented that bilingual children's lexical knowledge and progression are influenced by the level of exposure to each of their two languages and appear distinct from those of monolingual children (Gathercole, 2002a, 2002b, 2002c, 2007a, 2007b; Oller & Eilers, 2002a, 2002b). The timing of development is distinct (Gathercole, 2007; Gathercole & Hoff, 2007; Oller & Eilers, 2002b) and the distribution of knowledge is distinct (Cobo-Lewis et al., 2002; Grosjean, 1998; Oller, 2005; Oller & Pearson, 2002; Oller et al., 2007). Many have argued that these facts are relevant to the assessment and interpretation of linguistic performance of bilingual children: a child in the process of acquiring two languages will necessarily perform differently, at least at some points in the developmental process, from monolingual peers. Researchers have argued against the blind use of tests designed for monolingual children for evaluating bilingual children (e.g. Genesee & Nicoladis, 1995; Patterson, 1998; Pearson et al., 1993; Pearson, 1998), and researchers are gradually incorporating factors related to level of exposure to each language into the norming of standardized tests for bilinguals (e.g. Brownell, 2000a, 2000b; Cenoz & Gorter, in preparation; Dunn et al., 1997; Gathercole & Thomas, 2007; Gathercole et al., 2008, in press; Mattes, 1995; Munoz-Sandoval et al., 2005; Munro et al., 2005; O'Toole, this volume; Paradis & Libben, 1987; Verhoeven & Vermeer, 1993). What is less known is the enduring effect of differential exposure on the ultimate attainment of lexical knowledge in bilinguals.

The relationship between the bilingual's two languages is also gaining increasing attention in considerations of language assessment in bilinguals. The issue of whether bilingual children can show acceleration in grammatical development by bootstrapping from one language to another, or taking advantage of a structure learned in one language to gain a command of a similar structure in the other language, is of considerable ongoing debate (see Gathercole et al., in press).

The comparable issue in relation to the lexicon is whether children can show bootstrapping from one language to the other when there is a lexical similarity. Such a similarity might be, firstly, semantic, involving 'conceptual pairs' (e.g. *libro* and *book* refer to the same type of entity). There is considerable debate as to how best to 'count' such conceptual pairs in bilingual children's lexical repertoires; at least for some purposes, one may wish to measure a child's conceptual vocabulary, counting such items as 'one' (e.g. Méndez

Pérez *et al.*, 2010; Pearson *et al.*, 1993; Pearson, 1998; Umbel *et al.*, 1992; Umbel & Oller 1994). We will not focus here on that type of similarity, but instead on similarities involving both semantics and form, i.e. cross-language cognates, such as *camel* and *camello*, or borrowings from one language to the other, such as *armada*. One key question is whether bilingual children take advantage of such cognates or borrowings in learning words; for example, is it easier for a Spanish–English bilingual child whose dialect uses *carro* for 'car' to learn *car* in English than it is for a Spanish–English bilingual child whose dialect uses *coche* for 'car'? Is it easier for a Spanish–English bilingual child to learn *trumpet* in English, because of *trompeta*, than it is to learn *bear*, which corresponds to an unrelated form, *oso*? If so, we might expect bilingual children and adults to perform better on cross-language cognates than they do on non-cognates.

A second key issue has to do with assessment itself. A vocabulary test by force entails a 'sampling' of the individual's lexical knowledge. That sampling could, in principle, be designed to either include or exclude cross-language cognates. What are the benefits for one approach versus the other? On the one hand, knowledge of all words is relevant to any speaker's command of the language, so cognates are part of that overall knowledge. On the other hand, if a person tested in language A can 'guess' the meaning of a word in A because it sounds like a similar word in their stronger language B, then the performance could misrepresent that person's overall knowledge of language A.

Whether we include cognates in a test for bilinguals might depend on a number of factors. One is the relationship between the two languages themselves and the extent of the bilingual population who speaks those two languages. If the languages are unrelated or distant, the occurrence of cognates on a test may be unproblematic (but see the discussion below in relation to 'intuitive' cognates). When there is an extensive bilingual population (e.g. Welsh–English in Wales or Basque–Spanish in the Basque Country), however, there tends to be considerable borrowing between the two languages. The prevalence of cognates is particularly high in such long-standing language contact situations or when languages share etymological roots (e.g. Spanish and English). In the case of Spanish and English, cognates 'account for one-third to one-half the average educated person's active vocabulary' (Nash, 1997: viii). In a case like this, it may be desirable to avoid cognates in such tests, especially in a test for the minority language. For example, in the development of the *Prawf Geirfa Cymraeg*, a receptive vocabulary measure for Welsh bilingual children, Gathercole and Thomas (2007) opted to avoid cross-language cognates, so that children could not rely solely on English in order to perform well on Welsh words, even though there are numerous English borrowings used as standard words in Welsh.

A second consideration is whether or not there is evidence in fact from bilingual children's or adults' linguistic behavior showing differential performance on cognates versus non-cognates. If there is no difference in performance, then the issue is hypothetical only. However, if there is a difference in performance, then serious consideration must go into the question of their inclusion or exclusion. The jury is still out on this: García (1991) reported that 4th-grade Spanish/English bilinguals seldom made use of cognate knowledge while reading. She suggested that a certain level of development and possibly explicit instruction in the use of cognates was needed for bilinguals to adopt this strategy. On the other hand, Nagy *et al.* (1993) found that first-language vocabulary knowledge and ability to recognize cognates affected the performance of children of grades 4–6 in a comprehension task that included cognates. Méndez Pérez *et al.* (2010) conducted a study looking into vocabulary knowledge of Kindergarten and 1st-grade children and found that children who were dominant in Spanish performed better with cognates than with non-cognates, while children who were dominant in English performed better with non-cognates.

These issues with regard to cognates are not trivial. Apart from the theoretical issues involved, the common practice of developing tests by translating from one to another may exacerbate the issues, if this leads to a high occurrence of cognates on the tests (as we will see below for the PPVT and the TVIP).

Study 1

In order to address these questions, we conducted a study of vocabulary knowledge in end-state bilinguals in the Miami area. This study was part of a series of larger studies for which vocabulary measures were obtained for baseline information on the bilinguals' knowledge of the two languages. We report here on participants' performance on two standardized receptive vocabulary measures, the PPVT and the TVIP. Their performance relative to each other and to monolinguals is reported, as well as both 'external' and 'internal' factors that potentially influence performance.

Method

Participants

For this study we recruited 75 English–Spanish bilinguals living in South Florida. All participants had at least some tertiary education; that is, some were currently students at a university or college and some had already graduated. Their mean age was 22;6 (age range: 18–30 years) and 18 of them were women. Most of our participants (45%) identified their heritage background as Cuban, with others mentioning other Spanish-speaking Caribbean countries (11%), Central America (12%), South America (21%) and more than one heritage origin (11%). Additionally, for comparison purposes, we recruited a group of 25 monolingual Spanish speakers in Caracas, Venezuela, and another group of 25 monolingual English speakers in Sarasota, Florida. Participants in Venezuela were all 18-year-old first-year university students with very little or no knowledge of English (17 were women). Participants in Sarasota had a mean age of 33 years (age range: 18–61 years; 19 were women) and had very little or no knowledge of Spanish.

Bilingual participants were divided into groups according to their self-report of early childhood language exposure from their parents before entering first grade – that is, up to the age of 6 years. Each group consisted of 25 participants and were defined as follows:

- English and Spanish at home (ESH). These participants were born in the United States and had a relatively balanced input from parents in early childhood (between 40% and 60% input in each language).
- Only Spanish at home (OSH). These participants were born in the United States, but heard mostly Spanish (80% or more) input from their parents in early childhood.
- Early L1 Spanish–L2 English learners (L1S-L2E). These participants were born in a Spanish-speaking country but migrated to the United States between the ages of 2 and 12 years (mean age at time of migration = 4;6).

The ESH group had the largest proportion of US-born parents (24%), while very few of the parents for the OSH and L1S-L2E participants were born in the United States (2% and 6%, respectively). All individuals gave informed consent for participation, and they were paid for their participation. Each participant was also asked to complete an extensive background questionnaire, including questions about language usage inside and outside their homes at different ages, socio-economic indicators, attitudes towards each language, and so forth.

Materials

The PPVT and the TIVP were used. The tests consist of a series of words of increasing difficulty that are read out loud to participants in the presence of a plate with four drawings. The participant's task is to choose from these four drawings the one that corresponds best to the word heard. The initial point in the test is determined by the participant's chronological age, and testing continues until the administrator has determined baseline and ceiling levels for the participant. The raw vocabulary score is calculated by subtracting the number of errors from the ceiling level. A normed score can then be obtained by looking up this raw score in the corresponding age-appropriate table in the test's manual (see Dunn & Dunn, 1997, for a more in-depth description of the tests and scoring procedures). The PPVT is normed from ages 2 to 99 years, while for the TVIP all adults aged 18 years and above are grouped into the same norms. Due to this divergence in norming practices, in this chapter we will use raw scores from each test.

Procedure

Each participant was tested individually on the PPVT-4 and the TVIP-H by a bilingual researcher using the standard procedures of test administration described in Dunn and Dunn (2007) and Dunn et al. (1986), respectively. The PPVT and the TVIP were administered in one session, with order of presentation alternating between participants. The tests were separated by other unrelated experimental tasks that lasted approximately half an hour. In the tests, the experimenter read out loud each word and showed the participant four drawings on a plate. The participant then indicated which of the drawings corresponded best with the word read by pointing at it or stating the corresponding number.

Results

General performance on English and Spanish

Table 7.1 shows the mean raw scores for each bilingual group, and for the corresponding monolinguals, for the two languages. (Note that the maximum possible score for the PPVT is 228, while for the TVIP it is 125.) Table 7.2 shows the distribution of participants according to their performance within the norm for each test, more than one standard deviation below that norm, or more than one standard deviation above that norm.

On average, all groups scored higher than the norm on both languages, and all participants scored within 2 standard deviations from the norm. Table 7.2 shows that the distribution of vocabulary scores for all groups was skewed towards the right, with most participants in every group scoring within or above 1 standard deviation from the norm. This means that, in general terms, the bilingual groups reached an end-state in both languages that is comparable with the levels of their monolingual counterparts.

Within-language analyses of variance examining performance across groups revealed that there is no significant difference for English scores between any of the groups ($F(3, 96) = 0.85$, $p = 0.47$); that is, all bilingual

Table 7.1 Raw scores for the PPVT (English) and TVIP (Spanish) receptive vocabulary tests for each language background group

	PPVT – English (S.D.)	TVIP – Spanish (S.D.)
Mon ENG	207 (12.5)	–
ESH	205 (11.2)	110 (10.6)
OSH	203 (18.2)	111 (12.4)
L1S-L2E	208 (9.8)	117 (6.7)
Mon SPAN	–	118 (4.5)
NORM[a]	196	106

[a]This is the raw score that corresponds to a normed score of 100 at 17 years 11 months of age in each of the tests.

Table 7.2 Number of participants (out of 25 per cell) with vocabulary scores within the norm, more than 1 S.D. above the norm or more than 1 S.D. below the norm

	PPVT – English			TVIP – Spanish		
	Participants below 1 S.D. from the norm	Participants within 1 S.D. of the norm	Participants above 1 S.D. from the norm	Participants below 1 S.D. from the norm	Participants within 1 S.D. of the norm	Participants above 1 S.D. from the norm
Mon ENG	0	11	14	–	–	–
ESH	0	13	12	2	20	3
OSH	4	14	7	6	16	3
L1S-L2E	0	16	9	0	17	8
Mon SPAN	–	–	–	0	9	16

groups perform equivalently. On the face of it, then, there are no general lasting effects as a result of early language experience. (But see further analyses below taking exposure variables into account.)

In Spanish, on the other hand, an analysis of variance revealed two distinct homogeneous sets: Set 1 includes the Monolingual Spanish ($M = 118.01$; S.D. = 4.4) and L1S-L2E ($M = 117.4$; S.D. = 4.8) groups (with Scheffe correction for multiple comparisons $p > 0.99$), and Set 2 includes the ESH ($M = 109.9$; S.D. = 9.01) and the OSH ($M = 108.5$; S.D. = 14.4) groups (with Scheffe correction for multiple comparisons $p > 0.96$). The members of Set 1 showed a significantly better performance on Spanish vocabulary than members of Set 2 ($F(3, 96) = 7.47$; $p = 0.000$). This suggests that the greater exposure of the L1S-L2E group to Spanish has given them an advantage over the other bilingual groups in Spanish. It is interesting and important to note that the OSH group reported that they received Spanish almost exclusively up to about age 4;6, which is the average age of arrival into the United States for the L1S-L2E group. This indicates that the differences across the bilingual groups cannot be attributed to any possible differences in timing of their early exposure to Spanish.

These general results indicate that all groups seem to arrive at similar levels in English, but not in Spanish (even though they are all above the norm). It is interesting to note that the L1S-L2E group has the same score as the Spanish monolinguals, even though they did not receive formal education in Spanish above age 12 (which is the latest that any member of this group arrived in the United States). (There may, of course, be differences in domains that go beyond those tested in the receptive vocabulary measured through the Peabody inventory.)

The influence of 'external' factors

In order to examine the influence of external factors on bilingual participants' performance in Spanish and English, we entered information from the questionnaires into correlational analyses. That information included: (a) which language(s) the participants' parents spoke to them at different ages; (b) which language(s) older and younger siblings, as well as other adults, spoke to them; (c) which language(s) the participant spoke *to* parents, older siblings, younger siblings, and the like; and (d) parents' educational backgrounds.

Before examining the correlational analyses, it is worth commenting initially on the first three of these. Firstly, with regard to (a), Figure 7.1 shows the percentage of input from parents in Spanish (versus English) at different ages. The scores show two interesting factors: (i) relative differences between the groups in the prevalence of Spanish in input from the parents remain roughly constant through development – that is, the group with the most input in Spanish is the L1S-L2E group, next most in the OSH group, and the least in the ESH group; (ii) there is a steady decrease in Spanish input with age for all groups, particularly for the US-born participants (ESH and OSH groups). Note, however, that current parental Spanish input is roughly equivalent to the level at the start of puberty, suggesting a stabilization of language usage patterns at home.

With regard to (b), Table 7.3 shows the overall language input, with percentages shown for Spanish, from other members of the family during childhood. For the ESH group, Spanish input from both older and younger siblings is equally low, while for the other two groups we see that younger siblings tended to speak less Spanish to participants (cf. Bridges, 2009). Input from other adults (mostly grandparents, as reported by participants) is overwhelmingly in Spanish for all bilingual groups.

Finally, in relation to (c) above, Table 7.4 shows the percentage use of Spanish by the participants to others in various contexts. A series of ANOVAs

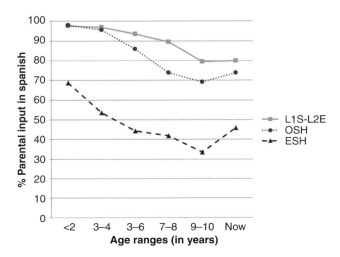

Figure 7.1 Trajectory of parental Spanish input at different ages

Table 7.3 Percentage input in Spanish (versus English) from other family members for each group of bilinguals

	From older siblings	From younger siblings	From adults (not parents)
ESH	7.3	10.0	90.0
OSH	34.4	23.3	94.5
L1S-L2E	74.2	65.5	94.3

Table 7.4 Percentage output by participants in Spanish (versus English)

	To parents	To older siblings	To younger siblings	Inside the classroom	Outside the classroom	To friends in school	To siblings now	To friends now
ESH	39.2	18.0	11.4	5.2	15.2	6.8	5.4	9.6
OSH	72.0	37.5	25.5	4.8	21.2	11.6	14.7	16.4
L1S-L2E	91.2	57.3	63.3	26.4[a]	43.6[a]	38.4[a]	30.0	20.0

[a]Note that many of the L1S-L2E participants attended at least part of elementary school in their countries of origin.

were conducted to examine the input and use of Spanish in distinct contexts across the three groups of bilinguals. An analysis of variance examining the language spoken to parents showed significant differences by group in the amount of Spanish spoken to their parents (F (2, 72) = 30.6, p = 0.000). All three groups differed significantly (with Scheffe correction for multiple comparisons, all p values <0.01). There was also a significant effect for Spanish output to older siblings (for the ones who had them) when growing up (F (2, 43) = 5.9, p = 0.01) and for current use of Spanish with siblings (F (2, 61) = 4.4, p = 0.016), with the L1S-L2E group using more Spanish than the ESH group (p < 0.05) but no significant differences otherwise. Findings for Spanish output to younger siblings (F (2, 34) = 10.2, p = 0.000), inside the classroom (F (2, 72) = 5.8, p = 0.005), outside the classroom (F (2, 72) = 5.6, p = 0.005), and to friends in school (F (2,72) = 8.8, p = 0.000) showed significant effects, with L1S-L2E using more Spanish than the other two groups (all p values <0.05), but no significant differences between the OSH and ESH groups. There were no significant differences across groups for current use of Spanish with friends.

Overall, then, we see that language production patterns by the participants themselves mirror those in the parental input, the L1S-L2E group speaking more Spanish than the other two groups in most contexts. The difference in Spanish usage between the OSH and the ESH groups is most noticeable in the context of the family, but not so much outside the home (i.e. school and friends). Importantly, all participants, even those from the L1S-L2E group, used less than 50% Spanish outside the home, and all of them speak less Spanish at present than earlier on with their peers (siblings and friends). Together, these data indicate that interaction with older family members 'anchors' the usage of Spanish at home, while interactions with peers or younger relations tend to occur in English.

A series of correlational analyses indicated some interesting relationships between vocabulary scores and such external factors. First, vocabulary scores for English correlated with the proportion of English used to interact with older siblings (for those who had them), both in terms of the language the older sibling spoke to them ($r = 0.41$, $p < 0.01$) as well as the language they spoke to the older siblings ($r = 0.35$, $p < 0.01$). Although these correlations do not indicate causality, we can speculate as to the source of the relationships between factors. In bilingual homes, older siblings are an important factor in introducing the majority language to the rest of the family (Bridges & Hoff, 2008), with younger siblings less likely to achieve proficiency in the minority language.

In contrast, Spanish vocabulary scores have a marginal negative correlation with the proportion of English used by parents throughout the participants' early childhood, especially at the earliest ages (age < 2: $r = -0.21$, $p = 0.07$; ages 2–4: $r = -0.22$, $p = 0.06$) and in the years prior to puberty (ages 9–12: $r = 0.22$, $p = 0.06$). As we saw above, the main source of Spanish for these bilinguals as they were growing up was in the home. Any reduction in the use of Spanish in favour of English appears to have affected their Spanish.

In addition, vocabulary scores correlated to some extent with parental education. English scores correlated with parental education for the ESH group ($r = 0.53$, $p < 0.01$), which is consistent with previous research (Oller & Eilers, 2002b), indicating that children from higher SES levels show higher scores in English. However, our results do not show this same relationship between English scores and parental education in the case of the OSH or the L1S-L2E groups. It is possible that these parents do not know enough English for them to choose to use it, even for high SES families.

At the same time, Spanish scores for the ESH group also show a positive correlation with parental educational level ($r = 0.41$, $p < 0.05$). Our speculation is that it takes effort to keep a bilingual home bilingual, and it is possible that higher SES families have more resources to make this happen. ESH families of higher SES may also attribute a higher value to keeping their children bilingual. Conversely, for the L1S-L2E group, there was a negative correlation between Spanish scores and parental education ($r = -0.45$, $p < 0.05$). It is possible that parents with a higher SES in this group attribute a higher value to language integration to the majority language. There was no significant relationship between these variables for the OSH group.

In sum, the influence of these external factors on performance on the vocabulary tests in English and Spanish appears to be as follows. There is a decreasing trend with age in parental Spanish input for all bilingual groups; this then stabilizes between early puberty and adulthood. In general, bilinguals tend to speak more Spanish to older members of their environment (parents, older siblings, other adults) and overwhelmingly more English with their peers. Also, there seems to be a zero sum game in terms of Spanish/English input from family members, where more usage of English seems to be associated with higher English scores but lower Spanish scores. In terms of socio-economic status (SES), higher SES is associated with higher Spanish scores for the ESH group, but the opposite is true for the L1S-L2E group.

The influence of 'internal' factors involving the relationship between the two languages – linguistic cognates

In order to explore whether knowledge of one language boosts the knowledge of the other, we examined performance on the tests more closely. An initial set of analyses revealed that scores on the two tests were highly correlated (ESH: $r = 0.75$, $p < 0.01$; OSH: $r = 0.62$, $p < 0.01$; L1S-L2E: $r = 0.53$, $p < 0.01$). It seems that the more balanced the input during childhood, the higher the correlation between the scores. However, the best explanation and interpretation for these correlations could have to do with the lexicon itself or with some other factor, such as cognitive level (see Gathercole *et al.*, 2013; in press). More informative perhaps is participants' performance on cognates versus non-cognates.

In order to assess the performance of these bilingual adults on words that are cognates in English and Spanish, we first examined the words on the PPVT and the TVIP to classify the words as cognates or non-cognates in the two languages. For the purpose of this study, we classified a cross-language word pair as 'linguistic' cognates if they were translation equivalents and shared at least three phonemes (as for *trumpet* and *trompeta*).

As pointed out by Méndez Pérez *et al.* (2010), several widely used vocabulary tests include a large percentage of Spanish–English cognate pairs – for example, the *Receptive One-Word Picture Vocabulary Test* (Brownell, 2000b) consists of more than 50% cognates for items intended for 6-year-old children, and cognates make up over one-third of the items in the picture section of the *Comprehensive Receptive and Expressive Vocabulary Test* (Wallace & Hammill, 2002). Looking specifically at the PPVT and the TVIP, we find that a large proportion of items in those tests can be classified as linguistic cognates. And the proportion tends to increase as the tests progress towards more difficult words: in English there is a higher presence of Germanic words in the lower registers and a higher presence of Latinates in the higher registers.

Differences in word frequency between the members of a cognate pair in their respective languages may affect whether one of them can assist in the recognition of the other or not. Of the 77 cognates present in the last 10 blocks of the PPVT, 31 have a higher frequency in Spanish than in English,[1] while only 16 have a higher frequency in English than in Spanish. We might therefore expect more influence going in the direction from Spanish to English than vice versa in vocabulary scores for bilinguals (cf. Hancin-Bhatt & Nagy, 1994).

For each participant, we calculated the accuracy rates separately for cognates and non-cognates on the two tests. The analyses here will focus on the English test, the PPVT, because there was a more even distribution of cognates to non-cognates among the words tested; on the TVIP, for the vocabulary range appropriate for adult participants, there were not enough non-cognates to make a meaningful comparison. The accuracy rates were calculated for each participant within his or her respective vocabulary range – that is, the proportion of correct responses for each type of word between the participant's basal and ceiling levels, as determined according to the instructions for the administration of the PPVT. This means that some participants saw more words than others, and some saw words of a higher set than others. On average, participants saw a total of 41 cognates versus 33 non-cognates across all groups (ESH cognates mean = 39.4, range: 33–53; non-cognates mean = 31.6, range: 27–43; OSH cognates mean = 43.1, range: 20–62; non-cognates mean = 34.2, range: 16–46; L1S-L2E mean = 41.6, range: 33–66; non-cognates mean = 33.3, range: 27–54; Mon ENG cognates mean = 39.5, range: 21–47; non-cognates mean = 31.6, range: 15–38).

The mean performance on cognates and non-cognates is shown by the home language in Table 7.5. Monolingual English speakers showed the same level of correct responses for cognates and non-cognates ($F (1, 24) = 1.7$; $p = 0.20$). This is as expected, since for monolinguals all words function as 'non-cognates', because there is no other language with which any word can be linked. Bilinguals of all types, on the other hand, showed a small but very reliable advantage of about 10% in the accuracy rate for cognates over non-cognates (ESH: $F(1, 24) = 32.5, p < 0.001$; OSH: $F(1, 24) = 24.7, p < 0.001$; L2: $F(1, 24) = 24.0, p < 0.001$).

These results suggest that all these adult bilinguals have a greater knowledge in English of the words that function as cognates in Spanish and English than of those that do not function as cognates. That is, it is either the case that they have had an advantage in learning words that are cognates in the two languages during the acquisition process for English or that when performing on a test like this, they can rely to some extent on their knowledge of Spanish to decipher the meaning of cognates in English.

Table 7.5 Percentage of correct responses on cognates versus non-cognates on the PPVT (English)

	Cognates % correct (S.D.)	Non-cognates % correct (S.D.)
Mon ENG	78.1 (7.6)	75.4 (14.0)
ESH	78.9 (9.6)	67.1 (13.6)
OSH	79.6 (8.3)	69.2 (12.3)
L1S-L2E	81.9 (7.6)	70.6 (13.6)

These results indicate that the presence or absence of inter-language cognates on tests such as these has a modest but significant effect on the overall performance of the bilingual. This result contrasts with the results presented by Umbel et al. (1992); and Umbel and Oller (1994), but this difference can be explained by noting that the adults tested here were college educated; they have probably encountered more of the members of the cognate pairs than the children included in these studies (consistent with, for example, Malabonga et al., 2008). As stated by Méndez Pérez et al. (2010), the amount of exposure to each language may have an effect on whether bilinguals make use of cognates, and our results from highly skilled bilinguals may be showing the 'ceiling state' of that gradient. An alternative explanation is that the link between cognates is an emergent property of vocabulary knowledge, not one that is initially present. That is, it may be that, as speakers become more fluent and knowledgeable in both their languages, they build links between those two languages.

Study 2

Beyond linguistic cognates: 'Intuitive' cognates

The analyses above concerning linguistic cognates examined words that are known to be related in the English and Spanish languages according to an *a priori* definition of cognates; these analyses and results examined whether bilingual speakers are cognizant of that relationship and use it in learning or interpreting words in their two languages. The better performance on the linguistic cognates over the non-cognates suggests, in fact, that they are. However, it is also possible that even without much experience with one or the other of their languages, a bilingual learner may be able to intuit relations between words that appear similar. If so, even without much knowledge of language A, speakers may be able to infer relations between words in language A with words in their other language, B, and perform well simply by making such inferences. At the same time, it is possible that words that would be classified as cognates following a rule-based definition such as the one above are not detected as such by a bilingual. This could happen, for example, because the bilingual does not know the corresponding word in language B (this is particularly likely if word frequency is much lower for the member of the pair in language B than in language A), or because the pronunciation is very different – for example, if there is a change in stress (e.g. *pentagon* vs. *pentágono*). If the purpose of using these instruments is to assess 'pure' knowledge of English, it may not be enough to look at linguistic cognates. Ultimately our goal is to discover what might make certain words 'easier' for a learner simply by virtue of their similarity to words in the bilingual's stronger language. On the other hand, if a cognate is not regularly recognized as such, any putative benefit derived from knowledge of the other language would not take effect.

In a follow-up study, we attempted to identify whether 'intuitive' cognates, or words that a learner might be able to 'guess' the meaning of because of similarity to a native-language word, might play a role in performance on vocabulary tests like these. We tested a set of naïve speakers (i.e. speakers who do not know English) in order to determine whether there were words whose meanings they were able to guess at better than chance level. We then reanalysed the Miami data to determine if such 'intuitive' cognates might have played a role in the bilinguals' performance.

Method

For this study, we collected data from monolingual Spanish speakers ('raters') and asked them to identify the items in the PPVT, that is, the *English* vocabulary test.

Participants: Raters

The raters were students at Universidad de Murcia (Spain) who reported their level of knowledge of English as 'minimal'; that is, they did not know more than a few words in English. In total, there were 30 participants (of which 22 were women) with an average age of 22;6 (range 18–31). All participants were students taking psychology classes at Universidad de Murcia, Spain, and they received extra credit for their participation.

Procedure

Participants heard recordings in English of the last 120 words of the PPVT in random order and were asked to select one of the corresponding four pictures from the PPVT as their response for each word they heard. Words were recorded by a native English speaker and were presented to participants over headphones. After giving their response, they were asked to indicate whether their response was the product of a random guess or not.

Results

We selected the words for which at least 50% of these monolinguals selected the right answer (random guesses were not counted towards this total), and labelled them as 'intuitive' cognates. The complete list is shown in Appendix A, with the corresponding Spanish words. There were four words that do not share three phonemes with their translation equivalents (*valley/valle, hatchet/hacha, polluting/contaminar, garment/prenda*), but were still recognized by more than 50% of the Spanish monolingual raters. The members of the first two pairs share sounds that are similar to each other, despite not being the same phonemes, while for the last two pairs, the English words are often borrowed in certain dialects of Spanish.

Table 7.6 Proportion of correct intuitive and rule-based/linguistic cognates

	Intuitive cognates % correct (S.D.)	Rule-based/linguistic cognates % correct (S.D.)
Mon ENG	76.9 (15.2)	74.4 (13.0)
ESH	80.7 (8.8)	74.6 (12.9)
OSH	82.0 (10.1)	74.2 (12.6)
L1S-L2E	83.2 (9.5)	76.2 (10.2)

More interestingly, there were 27 words (out of the 77 that were classified as cognates in Study 1 of this chapter based on a rule-based definition) that did *not* reach this 50% threshold; that is, 27 linguistic cognates were not recognized for their relationship with the corresponding Spanish words. These are shown in Appendix B, with the corresponding Spanish words.

Table 7.6 compares accuracy rates of the 50 cognates that *are* also intuitive cognates with the 27 rule-based/linguistic cognates. Monolingual English speakers showed the same level of correct responses for intuitive cognates and linguistic cognates (F (1, 24) = 0.7; $p = 0.39$). Bilinguals of all types, on the other hand, showed a small but significant advantage in the accuracy rate for intuitive over rule-based/linguistic cognates (ESH: $F(1, 24) = 5.5$, $p < 0.05$; OSH: $F(1, 24) = 14.4$, $p < 0.01$; L1S-L2E: $F(1, 24) = 9.0$, $p < 0.01$). Thus, bilinguals of all groups performed better with intuitive cognates than linguistic cognates that were not also intuitive cognates, suggesting that, in a fine-grained analysis, a rule-based categorization of the words does not capture the complexity of the issue. There was no difference between types of cognates for monolinguals, suggesting that the effect found for bilinguals is not due to intrinsic differences between the English words themselves. The differences in performance between the two groups of words are in all likelihood related to variations in the levels of phonological similarity across the pairs of words in the two languages. This suggests that further work on cognates in bilinguals' systems should differentiate distinct shades and types of cognates and their effects on bilinguals' performance.

General Discussion

Overall, we found that all groups of bilinguals achieved a high level of vocabulary knowledge in both languages, as measured by the Peabody receptive tests, and there is a high correlation between vocabulary scores in Spanish and English. This correlation could either be the result of an underlying language ability or, at least partially, arise from the interaction of knowledge of the two languages. The differences observed between the bilingual groups were mostly in relation to the minority language; that is, knowledge of vocabulary in English seemed to be 'topped up', even for groups that initially had little or no exposure to it (i.e. L1S-L2E, OSH), while the same was not true for Spanish (cf. Allen, 2006; Meisel, 2006; Schlyter & Hakansson, 1994; Treffers-Daller et al., 2007).

These results are consistent with the picture that emerges from responses to the language usage questionnaire, which revealed that Spanish usage decreased for all groups from the moment they entered school and continued to decrease at least until the early teen years. An interesting and novel finding is that the relationship between SES and vocabulary knowledge is not the same for all language background groups. While higher SES is associated with better Spanish knowledge for the ESH group, the opposite is true for the L1S/L2E group. In terms of the interaction of knowledge between the two languages, all bilingual groups seemed to make use of cognate information, showing a higher accuracy rate for cognates over non-cognates, at least in the direction from Spanish to English, as tested in this study. The influence of cognates in vocabulary assessment may depend on the specific composition of the test in question (some tests have more interlingual cognate pairs than others), the relative word frequency of the members of the cognate pair, and the age of the participants being tested (smaller children seem to be less able to use cognate information than older children and adults). In any case, it is an issue that deserves careful consideration in terms of the design of new vocabulary tests or the interpretation of results of existing ones, if they are to be administered to a bilingual population.

Finally, Study 2 showed that the interaction of language knowledge can go beyond what can be defined as cognates based on a simple definitional rule indicating a shared meaning and partial phonological overlap, as is common in language research. If one is to design a test of 'pure' vocabulary for a language, LA (i.e. aiming to avoid any influence from LB), it may be advisable to follow a similar approach to the one used in Study 2 for finding (and avoiding!) words that inherit some benefit from LB. On the other hand, the results of this study indicate that research into the influence of cognates may underestimate their effects if it includes word pairs that are not recognized as members of a cognate pair by a majority of participants.

Acknowledgements

This work is supported in part by ESRC & WAG/HEFCW Grant RES-535-30-0061, ESRC Grant RES-062-23-0175 and a WAG Grant on the Continued Development of Standardized Measures for the Assessment of Welsh, for which we are very grateful. We would like to thank research assistants Garamis Campusano and Jessica Miller for their work in recruiting participants and collecting the data, and Florida International University for their support. We are also grateful to Miami Dade College for its help in recruiting participants for this study, particularly to Dr Graciela Anrrich, Professor of ESL/Foreign Languages, for her assistance in recruitment and the logistics of testing, to Stephen Johnson and Dr Michelle Thomas for their personal support, and to the participants themselves. Also, thanks are due to Dr Miguel Pérez, Dr Rebecca Burns and Fraibet Aveledo for their assistance with the collection of monolingual Spanish and English data. This research would not have been possible without their collaboration.

Note

(1) Frequency counts for English were taken from the CELEX database (Baayen *et al.*, 1995), while for Spanish they were taken from LEXESP (Sebastián-Gallés *et al.*, 2000). Word frequencies were compressed using the formula log (1 + F), where log is the base 10 logarithm and F is the raw frequency in tokens per million. A member of a cognate pair was considered to have a higher frequency in one language than the other if between them there was a difference of frequency of at least 0.16 on the logarithmic scale; this difference is equivalent to the linear difference between 10 and 15 counts per million.

References

Allen, S. (2006) Language acquisition in Inuktitut–English bilinguals. Paper presented at Language Acquisition and Bilingualism: Consequences for a Multilingual Society, 4–7 May, Toronto.

Baayen, R.H., Piepenbrock, R. and Gulikers, L. (1995) *The CELEX Lexical Database* (CD-ROM). Philadelphia, PA: Linguistic Data Consortium, University of Pennsylvania.

Bates, E., Dale, P.S. and Thal, D. (1995) Individual differences and their implications for theories of language development. In P. Fletcher and B. MacWhinney (eds) *Handbook of Child Language* (pp. 95–151). Oxford: Basil Blackwell.

Bates, E. and Goodman, J.C. (1997) On the inseparability of grammar and the lexicon: Evidence from acquisition, aphasia and real-time processing. *Language and Cognitive Processes* 12 (5/6), 507–584.

Bates, E. and Goodman, J.C. (1999) On the emergence of grammar from the lexicon. In B. MacWhinney (ed.) *The Emergence of Language* (pp. 29–79). Mahwah, NJ: Erlbaum.

Bates, E., Marchman, V.A., Thal, D., Fenson, L., Dale, P., Reznick, J.S., Reilly, J. and Hartung, J. (1994) Developmental and stylistic variation in the composition of early vocabulary. *Journal of Child Language* 21 (1), 85–124.

Bridges, K. (2009) The effect of older siblings on toddlers' bilingual experience and bilingual development. Paper presented at the SRCD Biennial Meeting, 25 April, Denver, CO.

Bridges, K. and Hoff, E. (2008) The role of siblings in the English language development of bilingual toddlers in the US. In H. Chan, E. Kapia and H. Jacob (eds) *A Supplement to the Proceedings of the 32nd Boston University Conference on Language Development*. http://www.bu.edu/bucld/files/2011/05/32-Bridges.pdf

Brownell, R. (2000a) *Expressive One-Word Picture Vocabulary Test: Spanish-bilingual Edition*. Novato, CA: Academic Therapy Publications.

Brownell, R. (2000b) *Receptive One-Word Picture Vocabulary Test: Spanish-bilingual Edition*. Novato, CA: Academic Therapy Publications.

Cobo-Lewis, A.B., Pearson, B.Z., Eilers, R.E. and Umbel, V.C. (2002) Effects of bilingualism and bilingual education on oral and written English skills: A multifactor study of standardized test outcomes. In D.K. Oller and R.E. Eilers (eds) *Language and Literacy in Bilingual Children* (pp. 64–97). Clevedon: Multilingual Matters.

Conboy, B.T. and Thal, D.J. (2006) Ties between the lexicon and grammar: Cross-sectional and longitudinal studies of bilingual toddlers. *Child Development* 77 (3), 712–735.

Conti-Ramsden, G. and Jones, M. (1997) Verb use in specific language impairment. *Journal of Speech, Language and Hearing Research* 40, 1298–1313.

Dale, P.S., Dionne, G., Eley, T.C. and Plomin, R. (2000) Lexical and grammatical development: A behavioural genetic perspective. *Journal of Child Language* 27 (3), 619–642.

Dunn, L. and Dunn, L. (1997) *Peabody Picture Vocabulary Test-Third Edition.* Circle Pines, MN: American Guidance Service.

Dunn, L.M. and Dunn, L.M. (2007) *Peabody Picture Vocabulary Test – III.* Circle Pines, MN: American Guidance Service.

Dunn, L.M., Dunn, L.M., Whetton, C. and Burley, J. (1997) *The British Picture Vocabulary Scale* (2nd edn). Swindon: NFER-Nelson.

Dunn, L.M., Padilla, L. and Dunn, L.M. (1986) *Test de Vocabulario en Imágenes Peabody.* Circle Pines, MN: American Guidance Service.

Fenson, L., Dale, P.S., Bates, E., Reznick, J.S., Thal, D.J. and Pethick, S.J. (1994) Variability in early communicative development. *Monographs of the Society for Research in Child Development* 59 (5), 1–173.

García, G.E. (1991) Factors influencing the reading test performance of Spanish-speaking Hispanic students. *Reading Research Quarterly,* 26, 371–392.

Gathercole, V.C.M. (2002a) Command of the mass/count distinction in bilingual and monolingual children: An English morphosyntactic distinction. In D.K. Oller and R.E. Eilers (eds) *Language and Literacy in Bilingual Children* (pp. 175–206). Clevedon: Multilingual Matters.

Gathercole, V.C.M. (2002b) Grammatical gender in bilingual and monolingual children: A Spanish morphosyntactic distinction. In D.K. Oller and R.E. Eilers (eds) *Language and Literacy in Bilingual Children* (pp. 207–219). Clevedon: Multilingual Matters.

Gathercole, V.C.M. (2002c) Monolingual and bilingual acquisition: Learning different treatments of *that*-trace phenomena in English and Spanish. In D.K. Oller and R.E. Eilers (eds) *Language and Literacy in Bilingual Children* (pp. 220–254). Clevedon: Multilingual Matters.

Gathercole, V.C.M. (ed.) (2007a) *Language Transmission in Bilingual Families in Wales.* Cardiff: Welsh Language Board.

Gathercole, V.C.M. (2007b) Miami and North Wales, so far and yet so near: Constructivist account of morpho-syntactic development in bilingual children. *International Journal of Bilingual Education and Bilingualism* 10 (3), 224–247.

Gathercole, V. and Hoff, E. (2007) Input and the acquisition of language: Three questions. In E. Hoff and M. Shatz (eds) *The Handbook of Language Development* (pp. 107–127). Oxford: Blackwell.

Gathercole, V.C.M., Pérez-Tattam, R. and Stadthagen-González, H. (in press) Bilingual constructions of two systems: To interact or not to interact? In E.M. Thomas and I. Mennen (eds) *Unravelling Bilingualism: A Cross-disciplinary Perspective.* Bristol: Multilingual Matters.

Gathercole, V.C.M. and Thomas, E.M. (2007) *Prawf Geirfa Cymraeg, Fersiwn 7-11.* (Welsh Vocabulary Test, Version 7-11). www.pgc.bangor.ac.uk

Gathercole, V.C.M., Thomas, E.M. and Hughes, E. (2008) Designing a normed receptive vocabulary test for bilingual populations: A model from Welsh. *International Journal of Bilingual Education and Bilingualism* 11 (6), 678–720.

Gathercole, V.C.M., Thomas, E.M., Roberts, E., Hughes, C. and Hughes, E.K. (2013) Why assessment needs to take exposure into account: Vocabulary and grammatical abilities in bilingual children. In V.C.M. Gathercole (ed.) *Issues in the Assessment of Bilinguals* (pp. 20–55). Bristol: Multilingual Matters.

Genesee, F. and Nicoladis, E. (1995) Language development in bilingual preschool children. In E. Garcia and B. McLaughlin (eds) *Meeting the Challenge of Linguistic and Cultural Diversity in Early Childhood Education* (pp. 18–33). New York: Teachers College Press.

Grosjean, F. (1998) Studying bilinguals: Methodological and conceptual issues. *Bilingualism: Language and Cognition* 1 (2), 131–149.

Hancin-Bhatt, B. and Nagy, W. (1994) Lexical transfer and second language morphological development. *Applied Psycholinguistics* 15, 289–310.

Jones, M. and Conti-Ramsden, G. (1997) A comparison of verb use in children with SLI and their younger siblings. *First Language* 17 (50), 165–193.

Malabonga, V., Kenyon, D.M., Carlo, M., August, D. and Louguit, M. (2008) and Development of a cognate awareness measure for Spanish-speaking English language learners. *Language Testing* 25, 495–519.

Mattes, L.J. (1995) *Bilingual Vocabulary Assessment Measure.* Oceanside, CA: Academic Communication Associates.

Meisel, J.M. (2006) The development of the weaker language in bilingual first language acquisition. Paper presented at Language Acquisition and Bilingualism: Consequences for a Multilingual Society, 4–7 May, Toronto.

Méndez Pérez, A., Peña, E.D. and Bedore, L.M. (2010) Cognates facilitate word recognition in young Spanish-English bilinguals' test performance. *Early Childhood Services* 4, 55–67.

Muñoz-Sandoval, A.F., Cummins, J., Alvarado, G. and Ruef, M.L. (2005) *Bilingual Verbal Ability Test.* Scarborough, ON: Thomson Nelson.

Munro, S., Ball, M.J., Muller, N., Duckworth, M. and Lyddy, F. (2005) The acquisition of Welsh and English phonology in bilingual Welsh-English children. *Journal of Multilingual Communication Disorders* 3, 24–49.

Nagy, W.E., García, G.E., Durgunoğlu, A.Y. and Hancin-Bhatt, B. (1993) Spanish-English bilingual students' use of cognates in English reading. *Journal of Literacy Research* 25, 241–259.

Nash, R. (1997) *NTC's Dictionary of Spanish Cognates: Thematically Organized.* Lincolnwood, IL: NTC.

Oller, D.K. (2005) The distributed characteristic in bilingual learning. In J. Cohen, K.T. McAlister, K. Rolstad and J. MacSwan (eds) *Proceedings of the 4th International Symposium on Bilingualism* (pp. 1744–1749). Somerville, MA: Cascadilla Press.

Oller, D.K. and Eilers, R. (2002a) Balancing interpretations regarding effects of bilingualism: Empirical outcomes and theoretical possibilities. In D.K. Oller and R. Eilers (eds) *Language and Literacy in Bilingual Children* (pp. 281–292). Clevedon: Multilingual Matters.

Oller, D.K. and Eilers, R.E. (eds) (2002b) *Language and Literacy in Bilingual Children.* Clevedon: Multilingual Matters.

Oller, D.K. and Pearson, B.Z. (2002) Assessing the effects of bilingualism: A background. In D.K. Oller and R.E. Eilers (eds) *Language and Literacy in Bilingual Children* (pp. 3–21). Clevedon: Multilingual Matters.

Oller, D.K., Pearson, B.Z. and Cobo-Lewis, A.B. (2007) Profile effects in early bilingual language and literacy. *Applied Psycholinguistics* 28 (2), 191–230.

Paradis, M. and Libben, G. (1987) *The Assessment of Bilingual Aphasia.* Hillsdale, NJ: Laurence Erlbaum.

Patterson, J.L. (1998) Expressive vocabulary development and word combinations of Spanish-English bilingual toddlers. *American Journal of Speech and Language Pathology*, 7 (4), 46–56.

Pearson, B.Z. (1998) Assessing lexical development in bilingual babies and toddlers. *International Journal of Bilingualism* 2, 347–372

Pearson, B.Z., Fernández, S. and Oller, D. K. (1993) Lexical development in bilingual infants and toddlers: Comparison to monolingual norms. *Language Learning* 43, 93–120.

Schlyter, S. and Hakansson, G. (1994) Word order in Swedish as the first language, second language and weaker language in bilinguals. *Scandinavian Working Papers in Bilingualism* 9, 49–66.

Sebastián-Gallés, N., Martí, M.A., Cuetos, F. and Carreiras, M. (2000) *LEXESP: Léxico Informatizado del Español*. Barcelona: Edicions de la Universitat de Barcelona.
Treffers-Daller, J., Ozsoy, A.S. and van Hout, R. (2007) (In)complete acquisition of Turkish among Turkish–German bilinguals in Germany and Turkey: An analysis of complex embeddings in narratives. *International Journal of Bilingual Education and Bilingualism* 10 (3), 248–276.
Umbel, V.M. and Oller, D.K. (1994) Developmental changes in receptive vocabulary in Hispanic bilingual school children. *Language Learning* 44 (2), 221–242.
Umbel, V., Pearson, B.Z., Fernández, M.C. and Oller, D.K. (1992) Measuring bilingual children's receptive vocabularies. *Child Development* 63 1012–1020.
Verhoeven, L. and Vermeer, A. (1993) *Taaltoets Allochtone Kinderen Bovenbouw [Language Tests for Minority Children]*. Tilburg, The Netherlands: Zwijsen.
Wallace, G. and Hammill, D.D. (2002) *Comprehensive Receptive and Expressive Vocabulary Test – Second Edition (CREVT-2)*. Austin, TX: Pro-Ed.

Appendix A: List of Cognates that are both Rule-Based Cognates and Intuitive Cognates

Digital-digital, disecting-disectar, predatory-predatorio, palm-palma, clarinet-clarinete, valley-valle, kiwi-kiwi, interviewing-entrevistar, pastry-pastelito, assisting-asistir, solo-solo, inflated-inflado, trumpet-trompeta, archaeologist-arqueólogo, coast-costa, injecting-inyectar, interior-interior, citrus-cítrico, florist-florista, reprimand-reprender, carpenter-carpintero, primate-primate, trasparent-transparente, parallelogram-paralelogramo, pillar-pilar, consuming-consumir, cornea-córnea, peninsula-península, detonation-detonación, cerebral-cerebral, perpendicular-perpendicular, submerging-sumergir, cultivating-cultivar, ascending-ascender, sternum-esternón, maritime-marítimo, incarcerating-encarcelar, incandescent-incandescente, confiding-confiar, mercantile-mercantil, filtration-filtración, trajectory-trayectoria, converging-convergente, coniferous-conífera, timpani-tímpanos, reposing-reposar, cupola-cúpula, dromedary-dromedario, legume-legumbre, lugubrious-lúgubre

Appendix B: List of Rule-Based Cognates that are not Intuitive Cognates

directing-dirigir, hydrant-hidrante, fragile-frágil, beverage-bebida, rodent-roedor, inhaling-inhalar, mammal-mamífero, demolishing-demoler, isolation-aislamiento, pedestrian-peatón, departing-partir, feline-felino, aquatic-acuático, sedan-sedán, constrained-constreñido, valve-válvula, pentagon-pentágono, porcelain-porcelana, syringe-jeringa, quintet-quinteto, convex-convexo, torrent-torrente, arable-arable, supine-supine, vitreous-vítreo, cenotaph-cenotafio, calyx-cáliz

8 Profiling (Specific) Language Impairment in Bilingual Children: Preliminary Evidence from Cyprus

Maria Kambanaros and
Kleanthes K. Grohmann

The aim of this chapter is to highlight some of the challenges associated with the differential diagnosis of specific language impairment (SLI) in bilingual children living in Cyprus. The focus of this inquiry into (a)typical, bilingual language development draws on preliminary empirical evidence as to how language impairment presents in bilingual children for whom one language spoken is Cypriot Greek. Overall, the reader will be informed on (i) how SLI manifests in bilingual children and (ii) the major clinical issues influencing the assessment and diagnosis of SLI in childhood bilingualism, (iii) in countries where the main spoken language is not only understudied and not codified or even officially acknowledged but (iv) is used in parallel with an official standard variety.

By Way of Introduction: Some Background to Bilingual SLI

This chapter presents issues pertinent to the profiling of bilingual children with specific language impairment (henceforth, SLI). We focus on bilinguals from the perspective of Cyprus, and we highlight some of the problems one faces when trying to ascertain the prevalence, and more specifically the diagnosis, of SLI and other language impairments in such a linguistically diverse and complex situation.

The research described has been carried out in the Greek-speaking Republic of Cyprus, a small country with a population of around 800,000, whose speakers are typically characterized as exemplifying diglossia (Arvaniti, 2006; Newton, 1972). The official language is Demotic Greek, usually referred to as 'Standard Modern Greek' by linguists, yet the local variety, Cypriot Greek, differs in many interesting and grammatically relevant ways. However, Cypriot Greek is not officially acknowledged as a bona fide linguistic system or codified in other ways (for example, it does not have its own orthographic system), and research on it is limited. It has until recently been neglected as a legitimate subject of linguistic investigation, either as a grammatical system or in relation to its acquisition and development by young children. This holds for typical language development (henceforth, TLD), as it does for atypically developing and language-impaired children, including the identification of a concrete profile of SLI in Cypriot Greek.

However, recognition of Cypriot Greek as having its own structural characteristics is needed in order to properly diagnose Greek Cypriot children with SLI. One route might be to compare young Cypriot children's two systems of Greek, the standard variety and the local dialect, and treat them as bi(dia)lectal or even bilingual children, or at least as monolingual children with an additional variety in their linguistic repertoire. We will return to this issue below (see also Grohmann & Leivada, 2012; Kambanaros *et al.*, 2013b; Rowe & Grohmann, 2012). It should be noted, however, that international research comparing mono- *and* bilingual development for SLI is surprisingly lacking, leaving the potential implications of bilingualism for children with language disabilities as an underexplored area. An exception is work by Johanne Paradis and her colleagues spanning the past decade investigating SLI in bilingual children residing in Canada who are speaker–hearers of English and French (e.g. Paradis, 2010).

Furthermore, the assessment of developmental language disorders in multiple languages is complex and time-consuming for all parties involved: the clinician, the child, the child's family, any interpreters, and other health- or education-related professionals, such as occupational therapists or teachers. Given the premise of evidence-based practice, speech language therapists (henceforth SLTs), the term used in many parts of Europe and synonymous with speech language pathologists, are required by parents, professional associations and policy makers to provide a justification for their clinical practices on the basis of existing rigorous research evidence. A clear-cut finding is that both languages must be effectively assessed to ensure diagnostic accuracy, including the identification of level(s) of breakdown (Kohnert, 2010). Nevertheless, fundamental issues that linger and make this task daunting are the unavailability of bilingual language measures or tests for different language combinations and the serious lack of evidence of effective treatment methods for bilingual children with SLI (see Thordardottir, 2010, for a discussion of the latter issue).

By comparing children with language impairment to their typically developing peers, we may be able to identify language-specific factors that are most vulnerable in language impairment (e.g. specific grammatical forms). Such structures that are difficult for children with impaired language may then be incorporated into both formal and informal measures of language assessment and later serve as targets in language therapy. By comparing performance across the two language pairs, the impact of SLI on each language for comprehension as well as spoken and written language production will allow us to determine the level of linguistic breakdown for each language.

Of major theoretical and clinical significance is the search for universal and especially language-specific clinical markers across languages and within languages, that is, language behaviors that reliably differentiate children with and without SLI. Not much attention has been paid to developing a separate definition of SLI for bilingual children, despite sound evidence for the following (Peña & Bedore, 2009):

(i)   over- as well as under-identification is higher for bilingual SLI than for monolingual SLI;
(ii) bilingual children with SLI can perform differently, and typically better, than monolingual SLI on language tasks;
(iii) typically developing children acquiring a second language and monolingual children with SLI have similar linguistic profiles irrespective of dissimilar input experiences and internal learning mechanisms.

Speech and language therapy in Cyprus

For Greek-speaking Cyprus, speech and language therapy/pathology is a newly developing academic discipline. The first four-year accredited program in Speech and Language Therapy was only recently established at the European University Cyprus in Nicosia (September 2009). As a consequence, in 2012 all 389 members (346 women and 43 men) of the Association of Registered Speech Pathologists in Cyprus have received professional academic education and training outside of Cyprus from at least 10 different countries and diverse institutions, most prominently (in order of prevalence) from Bulgaria, the United States, Greece, the United Kingdom and Russia.

Without wanting to discuss qualitative differences or political implications, this reality has two important negative connotations: (i) most SLTs did not get acquainted with the properties of the Greek language as part of their training and course syllabi; and (ii) most did not work with Greek-speaking clients during their supervised clinical practicum prior to returning to Cyprus. On both counts, we would like to add the serious knowledge gap for Cypriot Greek, but the situation is serious enough even if we put the dialect issue aside. As such, clinicians may have insufficient linguistic expertise on which to base their interventions, which in turn impacts on language therapy and service provision to (bilingual) children with SLI whose mother tongue is Greek (be it Standard Modern or Cypriot Greek).

Furthermore, in 2012, 58% of the SLTs in Cyprus work in private practices and 36% in the public sector (6% are currently not practicing), with the majority providing services to schools and only a handful of therapists working in hospitals. The association is a member of the Standing Liaison Committee of European Union Speech and Language Therapists and Logopedists, which represents practicing SLTs at national and European levels.

Not much is known about how SLTs diagnose SLI in pre- or primary school-aged children in the Republic of Cyprus. For the purpose of discovering the current assessment procedures and practices (e.g. clinical competence, experience, intuition), we have adapted into Cypriot Greek the questionnaire given to SLTs in Ireland on the same topic by Lyons *et al.* (2008). However, we have constructed additional questions of particular interest to our research practice, such as whether SLTs speak a second or third language, which languages (given their training abroad), and their proficiency in those languages (self-rating across the domains of comprehension, expression, reading and writing).

We are in the process of obtaining data from this questionnaire. Other examples of questions SLTs are asked to answer include factors they consider most important in diagnosing SLI in the areas of syntax, semantics, pragmatics and other areas (e.g. non-word repetition, family history, etc.), the measures or tests they use to diagnose SLI (whether they use translated tests from the country of their training, for example), what causes them to initiate the consideration of a diagnosis of SLI, and topics they consider important for facilitating the diagnostic process and outcome. We intend to have collated our first results later this year. Preliminary data (10% of responses) analyzed for the purpose of this chapter reveal that bilingual children with SLI are more prominent on SLT caseloads than monolingual children, and that bilingualism imposes a serious challenge to the diagnosis of SLI for speech therapists working in Cyprus. This is exacerbated by the absence of standardized assessment measures for Cypriot Greek and other languages.

Conducting research with bilingual families in Cyprus

The demographics of Cyprus have changed dramatically during the past two decades. With the demise of the Soviet Union, large numbers of ethnic Greek populations have left their Soviet homelands and found domicile in Greece, but also in Cyprus. In subsequent years, and with increased mobility within Europe, many more migrants have arrived, from a multitude of cultural, ethnic, national and especially linguistic backgrounds. While partially covered in national censuses through the listing of nationalities, the current number of practical bilingual families in Cyprus cannot even be estimated due to the lack of information. For this reason, it is important to get an accurate picture of participants in bilingual research on (a) TDL, including SLI.

When working with bilingual children in Cyprus, whether TLD or potential SLI, we first request that the parents complete a bilingual language history questionnaire. We are now in the fortunate position of having several questionnaire types at our disposal; these are described in brief below.

So far, we have adapted the L2 Language History Questionnaire (Li et al., 2006), available electronically, from its original English into Greek (accommodating both Cypriot Greek and Standard Modern Greek), Russian and Bulgarian. Parents of bilingual children who will participate in our research are requested to complete the questionnaire for their child (and themselves) prior to the commencement of testing in the language of their choice. The reported information concerns at what age and in what contexts languages were acquired, as well as estimating the child's (and their own) degree of proficiency based on language amount and contexts of use for each language. This information is essential for an understanding of the type of bilingualism, the combinations of languages, input, learning mechanisms and exposure.

In addition, we are currently devising – that is, adapting to Cypriot Greek and other aspects of language use in Cyprus – several alternative or complementary questionnaires. One prominent example is the biSLI Questionnaire (COST Action IS0804, 2009–2013), initiated by Laurie Tuller and colleagues, and essentially based on the Alberta Language Environment Questionnaire (Paradis et al., 2010). One advantage of this tool is quantitative comparability through the large dataset on bilingual children across Europe and beyond to be collected from the Action's many participants.

Another questionnaire-based project aims to design a usable version of the MacArthur–Bates Communication Development Inventory (CDI; Fenson et al., 1994). This will be an immensely important tool for tracking early language acquisition and development in toddlers and younger children, focused on but not restricted to vocabulary items (see Ezeizabarrena et al. in this volume and O'Toole in this volume). Our Cyprus CDI is designed in such a way as to discriminate between Cypriot Greek and Standard Modern Greek, and it can easily be extended to bona fide bilingual populations. With a sufficient number of participants, results obtained from this study will assist in the early diagnosis for language impairment based on the CDI's vocabulary profile, as has been implemented for other languages (see, for example, Skarakis-Doyle et al., 2009, for a recent study on English).

Diagnostic measures developed for bilingual SLI populations

In this section we report on the diagnostic measures developed by our research team for the assessment of SLI in bilingual Greek Cypriot children. The aim was to develop tools with predictive indices for language impairment. We are interested in identifying universal and language-specific clinical markers (i.e. language behavior that reliably differentiates children with and without SLI).

The Cypriot Greek Language Screening Tool for identifying at-risk preschoolers

The Cypriot Greek Language Screening Test (CGLST) was developed in the ongoing CySLI Project (http://www.research.biolinguistics.eu/CySLI), a large-scale research study aimed at the early identification of SLI in monolingual, bilectal children – namely, Greek Cypriot children who acquire Cypriot Greek and Standard Modern Greek. The CGLST is a screening tool that takes around 10 minutes to administer. Domains chosen for investigation were based on what have been identified in COST Actions A33 and IS0804 as strong markers for the identification of SLI across languages. Table 8.1 lists the domains screened using the CGLST.

The immediate scientific objective with obvious social and educational benefits of a screening tool is to determine the number of preschoolers with SLI before entering primary education. If one applies the prevalence figure reported for 5-year-old (monolingual) preschoolers with SLI in the United States (7%; Tomblin et al., 1997) to the number of preschoolers in Cyprus (2012: 9894; Cyprus Ministry of Education and Culture), then the potential number of children with SLI alone could be 700. What remains to be determined is how many of those children are bilingual. Bilingual children for the proposed research are children who are speakers of Cypriot Greek and a second language (e.g. Russian).

Children labeled 'at risk' after the screening stage will be assessed using the specific diagnostic tools reported in the section below for the (differential) diagnosis of SLI in both their languages (where possible). Results regarding the number of bilingual preschoolers presenting with SLI will help establish overall prevalence rates of SLI in the bilingual Greek Cypriot preschool population.

Tools for assessing SLI in Greek

Practically speaking, assessing for SLI in Greek Cypriot children is a new area of investigation initiated after the participation of our research group in COST Action A33. So far, a test battery has been composed comprising a number of tools to identify SLI in children based on the emerging data from three years of intensive testing on a large number of bilectal children with TLD and smaller groups of children with SLI. We are currently in the process of administering the normed tests on simultaneous or early sequential,

Table 8.1 Domains of language screened by the CGLST

Domain	Marker	Items
Lexicon	Confrontation naming	Stimulus question: 'What is this?' (10 fruits, high and low frequency)
Phonology	Articulation	Based on the child's naming responses
Phonology Working memory	Non-word repetition (based on Greek phonotactics)	6 items: one 3-syllable word, three 4-syllable words, two 5-syllable words
Morphosyntax Working memory	Sentence repetition	6 items: two sentences testing phonological memory (between 6 and 16 syllables) and four testing grammatical constructs (e.g. object relative clauses, *wh*-questions, negation)
Lexicon Semantics	Definitions	1 verb: 'Tell me all you know about "digging"'. 1 noun: 'Tell me all you know about "scissors"'
Lexicon Morphosyntax Pragmatics	Narrative re-tell	A short story (10 lines) that the child repeats after the examiner. Testing: coherence, production of syntactically correct sentences, use of pronouns, tense, vocabulary, etc. 2 mental verbs: *think, be scared*
Phonology Morphosyntax Working memory	Following commands	3 items: 'Put the pen under the chair and give me the pencil.' 'Show all the fruit *except for* the apple.' '*Before* you point to the pear, point to the cherries'
Phonology	Phonological discrimination	10 nonsense word pairs are produced by the examiner; the child has to say whether each pair sounds the same or different

typically developing bilingual children of (Cypriot) Greek–English and (Cypriot) Greek–Russian language backgrounds. The broader aim of this study is to measure how bilinguals with TLD perform on standardized tests created for (Greek) monolinguals, in order to see whether their performance would fall below the normal range of monolingual children with TLD (see Kambanaros & Karpava, 2012).

Past studies have shown that bilingual children with TLD often perform below monolingual age peers on standardized tests, with *over-identification of SLI in bilinguals* a potential outcome (see Kohnert, 2010, and references within). For this reason, the same tools are currently being used to pilot the identification of SLI in the (Cypriot) Greek language of bilingual children (as either L1 or L2). The tools can be divided into two types, linguistic and non-linguistic, as listed in Table 8.2. We also report the domains tested by each tool and note which tools are norm-referenced for Greek.

In addition, we are piloting a second group of language-specific tools to investigate the linguistic abilities of bilingual (potential) SLI children in both their languages for different linguistic skills and/or domains. The languages under investigation are (Cypriot and Standard Modern) Greek, English, Russian and Bulgarian, with additional extensions to Romanian in the near future. The language-specific tools are reported in Table 8.3 for each language under investigation.

Profiling the linguistic skills of bilingual children with SLI in Cyprus

Very few studies have investigated language impairment in Greek Cypriot children. One of the first and only studies outside the present research activities within the Cyprus Acquisition Team was that by Petinou & Terzi (2002), who report on naturally occurring spontaneous speech samples of five typically developing children and five children identified with SLI, all monolingual, in a longitudinal study in which data were collected every two months. Other studies have examined the speech acquisition patterns of late talkers and potential SLI children (Petinou & Okalidou, 2006) or the processing of mental state verbs by school-aged children confirmed with SLI (Spanoudis *et al.*, 2007). Recently, studies investigating the language performance of bilingual SLI compared to monolingual SLI children on various linguistic tasks are emerging, carried out by our research group.

In this section, we report two such studies. The first study focuses on lexical retrieval of action and object words, and the second on a narrative re-tell task. Both studies aim to decipher whether bilingual SLI children's performance patterns are parallel to those of children with TLD (monolingual/bilingual), or are parallel to those with (monolingual) SLI, or are distinct from both. The rationale behind each study is described in the introductions to Study 1 and Study 2.

Table 8.2 Diagnostic tools for Greek

Tool	Domain	Source
Linguistic		
Developmental Verbal Intelligence Quotient (DVIQ)[a]	5 subtests: • expressive vocabulary • comprehension of morphosyntax • production of morphosyntax • sentence repetition • comprehension of metalinguistic concepts	Stavrakaki and Tsimpli (2000)
Clitics-in-Islands Tool	Clitic production	COST Action A33 (2006–2010)
Binding Tool	Reflexives, pronouns/clitics	
Relative Clause Tool	Relative clause production	
Wh-Exhaustivity Tool	Comprehension of single and multiple wh-questions as well as exhaustivity	
Tense Tool	Comprehension of tense	
Aspect Tool	Comprehension of aspect	
Implicatures Tool	Quantifier domain selection	
Quantifier Tool	Distributive quantification	
Peabody Picture Vocabulary Test[a]	Receptive vocabulary	Simos et al. (2011)
Phonetic and Phonological Articulation Test[a]	Articulation and phonological processing	Panhellenic Association of Logopedists (1995)

(continued)

Table 8.2 (*continued*)

Tool	Domain	Source
Picture Word Finding Test[a]	Expressive vocabulary	Vogindroukas et al. (2009)
Athina Test of Learning Difficulties[a]	Learning abilities	Paraskevopoulos et al. (1999)
Cypriot Greek Word and Non-Word Repetition Test	Word repetition	Theodorou (in progress)
Cypriot Greek Sentence Repetition Tool	Sentence repetition	
Non-linguistic		
Raven Coloured Progressive Matrices (RCPM)	Non-verbal performance	Raven et al. (2000)
Tests of executive function	Shifting, inhibition	COST Action IS0804 (2009–2013)

[a]The tool is norm-referenced for Greek (SMG).

Table 8.3 Assessment measures used to investigate language impairment across languages and domains

	Cypriot Greek	Standard Modern Greek	English	Russian	Bulgarian
Lexical access for nouns and verbs	Cypriot Object and Action Test (COAT: Kambanaros et al., 2013a)	Greek Object and Action Test (GOAT: Kambanaros, 2003)	Greek Object and Action Test (English version: Kambanaros, 2003)	Russian Object and Action Test (ROAT; work in progress)	Bulgarian Object and Action Test (BOAT; work in progress)
Articulation and/ or phonological processing	Adaptation of the Phonetic and Phonological Articulation Test (Panhellenic Association of Logopedists, 1995)	Phonetic and Phonological Articulation Test (Panhellenic Association of Logopedists, 1995)	Goldman–Fristoe Test of Articulation (Goldman & Fristoe, 2000)		
Word-finding	Adaptation of the Word Finding Vocabulary Test (Vogindroukas et al., 2009)	Word Finding Vocabulary Test (Vogindroukas et al., 2009)	Word Finding Vocabulary Test (Renfrew, 1997)	Russian Language Proficiency Test for Multilingual Children (Gagarina et al., 2010)	Adaptation of the Word Finding Vocabulary Test (Vogindroukas et al., 2009)
Narratives	Adaptation of the Bus Story Test (Renfrew, 1997)	Adaptation of the Bus Story Test (Renfrew, 1997)	Bus Story Test (Renfrew, 1997)	Adaptation of the Bus Story Test (Renfrew, 1997)	Adaptation of the Bus Story Test (Renfrew, 1997)
Sentence construction	COAT, sentence construction subtest	GOAT, sentence construction subtest	English version of the GOAT, sentence construction subtest	ROAT, sentence construction subtest	BOAT, sentence construction subtest

(continued)

Table 8.3 (*continued*)

	Cypriot Greek	Standard Modern Greek	English	Russian	Bulgarian
Definitions	COAT, definition subtest	GOAT, definition subtest	English version of the GOAT, definition subtest	ROAT, definition subtest	BOAT, definition subtest
Action naming	Adaptation of the Greek version of the Action Picture Test (Vogindroukas et al., 2010)	Greek version of the Action Picture Test (Vogindroukas et al., 2010)	Action Picture Test (Renfrew, 1997)	Adaptation of the Greek version of the Action Picture Test (Vogindroukas et al., 2010)	Adaptation of the Greek version of the Action Picture Test (Vogindroukas et al., 2010)
Concepts (comprehension)			Boehm Test of Basic Concepts (Boehm, 2000)	Boehm Test of Basic Concepts (Boehm, 2000)	
Auditory comprehension	Adaptation of the Test of Receptive and Expressive Language Abilities (Vogindroukas & Grigoriadou, 2009)	Test of Receptive and Expressive Language Abilities (Vogindroukas & Grigoriadou, 2009)	Test of Auditory Comprehension of Language (TACL: Carrow-Woolfolk, 1999)	Test of Auditory Comprehension of Language (TACL: Carrow-Woolfolk, 1999)	
Other language functions		AnOmilo-4 (Panhellenic Association of Logopedists, 1995)	[a]		

[a]Clinical Evaluation of Language Function (CELF: Semel & Wiig, 1980); Verb Agreement and Tense Test (VATT: van der Lely, 1999); Test of Active and Passive Sentences – Revised (TAPS-R: van der Lely, 1996); Preschool Language Scale (Zimmermann et al., 2002); TROG-2 (Bishop, 2003).

Study 1: Bilingual Lexical Access for Action and Object Words

Introduction

Early research has shown that children with SLI are less accurate at naming pictures of common objects (nouns) than age-matched peers with no language impairment because of weakly differentiated and inadequately organized semantic representations (Lahey & Edwards, 1996, 1999). Lexical-semantic difficulties have been studied less in bilingual SLI but could potentially serve as a clinical marker that will vary less across languages (Bedore & Peña, 2008). Recently, monolingual (English-speaking) children with SLI were reported to have more difficulty retrieving action compared to object words (Sheng & McGregor, 2010). A similar dissociation with verbs or action names as the impaired class compared to noun or object names was described for bilectal Greek Cypriot children within our research group (Kambanaros et al., 2013b). In the case of bilingual SLI, if such a dissociation can be found, it would constitute evidence that grammatical category (verb and noun) *is* an organizing principle of the language system shared across languages (Miozzo et al., 2010). This has led to our assumption that verb–noun differences should be comparable across languages (Kambanaros & Grohmann, 2010; Kambanaros et al., 2010).

Aim

The aim of the study is to compare bilingual children with and without SLI with their monolingual counterparts on the same research tool. This line of research may shed light on the role of grammatical category in the organization of the bilingual lexicon. We predicted that bilingual children with SLI would have greater difficulty with lexical access for action and object words compared to their monolingual peers with SLI, given the availability of words (i.e. nouns and verbs) in two languages. Similarly, action words would be significantly more difficult to retrieve than object words, supporting the trend irrespective of language type reported so far in the literature.

Method

Participants

Five groups of children participated in this study:

(i) 30 monolingual children with TLD (15 girls, 15 boys), aged 6;0–6;11 years (6 years 0 months to 6 years 11 months) (mean: 6;3);

(ii) 10 younger children with TLD (2 girls, 8 boys) aged 3;5–5;2 years (mean: 4;4);

(iii) 14 monolingual children diagnosed with SLI (4 girls, 10 boys), aged 5;5–9;9 years (mean: 6;9);

(iv) 4 bilingual children diagnosed with SLI (2 girls, 2 boys), aged 6;6–8;10 years (mean: 7;4);

(v) 6 bilingual children with TLD (3 girls, 3 boys), aged 4;6–6;6 years (mean: 5;4).

The (monolingual and bilingual) children with SLI were recruited from SLTs in public primary education and/or therapists in private practice. All children were in mainstream education and in the school grade corresponding to their chronological age. Of the 18 children with SLI, 12 were receiving speech language therapy at the time of testing, three of these in special education services separate from their classmates and the regular classroom (i.e. pull-in/out service model). Subject selection inclusion criteria for both this and the following study included being either a Greek Cypriot with a monolingual background for the monolingual children or a bilingual child with Cypriot Greek as one of the languages spoken (either L1 or L2).

The TLD children were recruited randomly from three public primary schools and one Kindergarten in the Nicosia district after approval from the Ministry of Education and Culture and upon written parental consent. No child classified as TLD had received speech and language therapy or special education services.

Both groups of children with SLI were diagnosed prior to the research using a battery of norm-referenced tests for Greek (see Table 8.2) by two SLTs (one being the first co-author) as part of a larger investigation (Theodorou, in progress). Testing included measures of receptive and expressive morphosyntax, receptive and expressive vocabulary, and sentence recall from the Developmental Verbal Intelligence Quotient (DVIQ: Stavrakaki & Tsimpli, 2000). The SLI groups scored significantly lower than their age-matched peers on all language measures. Children's non-verbal performance was assessed using Raven's Coloured Progressive Matrices (Raven et al., 2000). The four simultaneous bilingual children with SLI came from the following language backgrounds: two are English, one is Romanian and the fourth is Arabic, with (Cypriot) Greek the other language for all four.

Case history information was obtained through the parents of all the children. For the bilingual groups, parents completed our bilingual language questionnaire (see section on 'Conducting research with bilingual families in Cyprus', above). No participating child (SLI or TLD) had a history of neurological, emotional or behavioral problems. All the children's hearing and vision were adequate for testing purposes, and they showed normal performance on screening measures of non-verbal intelligence or as reported by school psychologists. Moreover, the children showed normal articulation and had no gross motor difficulties. All children came from families with a medium to high socio-economic status as measured by mothers' education using the European Social Survey database (2010). Since mothers' education was measured on an ordinal scale, Kruskal–Wallis was used to examine for differences among the five groups. The result was significant, $\chi^2(4) = 14.41$, $p = 0.006$. Pairwise Mann–Whitney tests revealed that significant differences existed only between the monolingual SLI and the older TLD group ($z = -3.35, p = 0.001$) as well as the younger TLD group ($z = -3.43, p = 0.001$) groups. In both cases, the mothers' education level was lower for the monolingual SLI group.

The preschool TLD children serving as the language controls were matched with the SLI groups based on their scores on Vogindroukas et al.'s (2009) standardized Greek version of the Renfrew Word-Finding Vocabulary Test (Renfrew, 1997). Descriptive information about the background testing of participants is presented in Table 8.4.

Note that while we refer to Greek Cypriot children who only speak Greek as 'monolingual', they are in fact bilectal, to use the term reintroduced by Rowe and Grohmann (2012). That is, their native language is clearly Cypriot Greek (all participants come from Greek Cypriot family backgrounds), but with the onset of schooling and through media, they acquire as their second dialect or variety Standard Modern Greek (for more discussion, see also Grohmann & Leivada, 2012; Kambanaros et al., 2013a).

Materials

The Cypriot Object and Action Test (COAT), adapted by Kambanaros et al. (2013a) to Cypriot Greek from the original GOAT for Standard Modern Greek (Kambanaros, 2003), was administered to assess retrieval of object and action names. Thirty-five nouns and 39 verbs were elicited. The nouns were words for concrete objects; the verbs were words for everyday activities. All verbs were monotransitive with either simple internal word structures of [root + affix] or slightly more complex, with an additional suffix. All action names corresponded to either an instrumental verb, where an instrument is part of the action (e.g. cutting), or to a non-instrumental verb (e.g. climbing).

Nouns and verbs were matched for frequency (Mann–Whitney $z = -0.154, p = 0.878$), syllable length ($z = -0.610, p = 0.542$), age of acquisition ($z = -0.401, p = 0.688$), imageability ($z = -4.047, p = 0.00$), and picture complexity ($z = -2.644, p = 0.008$). Lemma frequencies for object and action names were calculated based on the printed word frequency count for Standard Modern Greek (Hatzigeorgiou et al., 2000); at this time, there are no word frequency data available for Cypriot Greek. Object words were significantly more imageable than action words. Similarly, action pictures were significantly more complex than object pictures (Kambanaros et al., 2013a).

Procedure

The object and action tasks were presented in one or two sessions. Testing was conducted in a quiet room at the school. Each child was tested

Table 8.4 Mean scores for participating groups on verbal and non-verbal subtests of the assessment battery for SLI

Test	Notes	TLD scores	SLI mean scores
Raven's matrices			85.4 mean standard score
DVIQ (morphosyntax production)	TLD scores: mean results of administering the test to 16 children aged 4;6–9;11	19.9	12.3
DVIQ (morphosyntax comprehension)		26.4	22.4
DVIQ (sentence repetition)		46.8	40.8
DVIQ (vocabulary)		22.3	15.7
DVIQ (metalinguistic abilities)		20.1	17.5
PPVT	TLD scores: mean results of administering the test to 10 children aged 4;8–9;11	79.3	69.3
Picture Naming Test	Norms (in SMG) for children aged 5;1–8;0	26.5–33.2	30.2 (S.D. 7.9) TLD scores for mean age 27.5
Bus Story Test (information)	TLD scores: mean results of administering the test to 11 children aged 4;6–9;11	29.8	23.3

Table 8.4 (*continued*)

Bus Story Test (A5LS)	8.8		6.5
Bus Story Test (subordinate clauses)	4.1		2.0
Bus Story Test (MLU)	5.1		3.8
Bus Story Test (sentences)	18.4		17.8
Athina Test (vocabulary definition)	9–32	Norms (in SMG) for children aged 5;4–9;10	15 (6;7) 16 (6;7) *TLD scores for mean age*
			8.3
Athina Test (sounds distinction)	14–28	Norms (in SMG) for children aged 5;4–9;11	20 (6;8) 21 (6;11) *TLD scores for mean age*
			17.6

individually. Children were asked to name the object or action represented in the photograph in a single word. Action names were required in the third person singular. Two examples were provided before testing. The stimulus question(s) were repeated once for children who did not respond. If no response was given, the item was scored as incorrect. No time limits were placed, and self-correction was allowed. Responses were recorded and transcribed verbatim by the first author and checked by the second.

Results

The percentages of correct responses were calculated for object and action names, and are shown in Figures 8.1 and 8.2, respectively. The bold line in the box plots represents the median, and the 'edges' of each 'box-and-whiskers' signify the maximum and minimum values. The dashed line was added to provide a comparison point to compare how the median bilingual SLI (and bilingual TLD) groups performed relative to the younger TLD children and the monolingual (bilectal) SLI and older TLD groups. (Note that they performed similarly to the former and worse than the latter in both cases.)

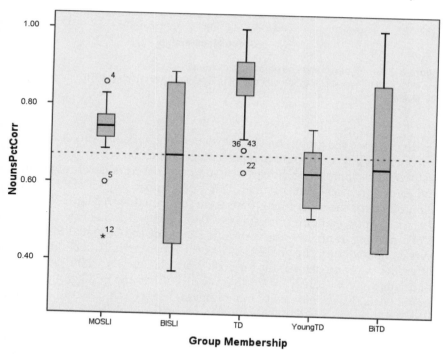

Figure 8.1 Group performances on object naming
Key: MOSLI, monolingual SLI; BISLI, bilingual SLI; TD, typically developing; BITD, bilingual typically developing.

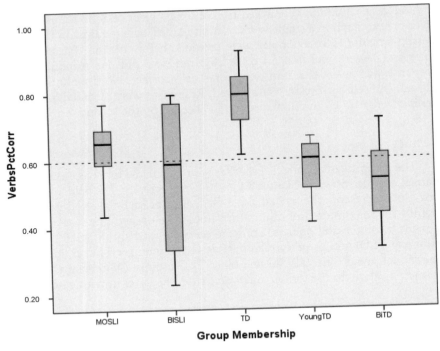

Figure 8.2 Group performances on action naming
Key: MOSLI, monolingual SLI; BISLI, bilingual SLI; TD, typically developing; BITD, bilingual typically developing.

To compare the groups on the two dependent variables simultaneously (percentage correct on nouns and percentage correct on verbs), a MANOVA test would be appropriate; however, assumptions of equality of covariances and error variances were not met. Pairwise comparisons of the bilingual SLI group with the other four groups were conducted with Mann–Whitney U tests, adopting a Bonferroni adjusted $0.05/3 = 0.017$ level of significance. When naming accuracies for verbs and nouns of the bilingual SLI group were compared with the performance of the monolingual SLI children, the difference was non-significant for both word classes ($z = -0.061$, $p = 0.951$ for nouns and $z = -0.122$, $p = 0.903$ for verbs). When the biSLI group (mean age 7;4 years) was compared to monolingual (henceforth, bilectal) children with TLD (mean age 6;3), there was no significant difference in performances for action ($z = -1.56$, $p = 0.120$) and object ($z = -1.67$, $p = 0.095$) words. Similarly, when the biSLI group was compared to younger bilectal TLD children (mean age 4;4), there was no significant difference in performances for action ($z = -0.284$, $p = 0.777$) and object ($z = -0.142$, $p = 0.887$) words. Finally, when the biSLI group was compared to younger bilingual

children with TLD (mean age 5;4), there was no significant difference in performances for action ($z = -0.476$, $p = 0.670$) and object ($z = -0.214$, $p = 0.831$) words. Generally, children with SLI *were* less accurate in (object and action) naming than both the age-matched and the younger children with TLD; however, for the biSLI group the differences *were* non-significant. This may suggest that children with SLI are delayed – but *not* atypical.

To summarize, the bilingual children with SLI (albeit four only) did not show a significant difference in naming accuracies for action and object names compared to their monolingual counterparts with SLI. In other words, the outcome of children with SLI learning two languages for verb and noun retrieval at the single-word level revealed no significant differences between the bilingual and monolingual SLI groups for the standard language Greek (see Kambanaros *et al.*, 2013b).

Study 2: Narrative Re-tell

Introduction

In this study (Theodorou & Grohmann, 2010), narrative samples were used to quantify language productivity and language impairment in monolingual and bilingual children using story re-tell. This is a pilot study; fully fledged results will be presented elsewhere (Theodorou, in progress). In addition, ongoing research as part of the Cyprus Acquisition Team's participation in COST Action IS0804 will compare telling with re-telling tasks and also consider other aspects of narrative abilities.

Aim

Narrative ability is one of the most promising ways to assess communicative competence in children: coordination of lexical, morphosyntactic, phonological and pragmatic elements is needed to produce narrations. Narratives might even serve as a diagnostic tool for SLI, since children with SLI are reported to have difficulties producing (oral) narratives (see Justice *et al.*, 2006). The aim of the study is to compare SLI children with their TLD peers to see whether there are qualitative differences in their re-tell abilities. We predicted that the impaired children would produce re-tell narratives less competently with respect to length, lexical diversity, sentence complexity and content, as has been reported in the literature (Gillam & Pearson, 2004). By adding a small group of older bilingual children with SLI, we wanted to see whether the impaired children improve in their narrative abilities over time or whether bilingualism plays a role.

Method

Participants

Three groups of children participated in this study:

(i)   12 monolingual children with TLD (7 girls, 5 boys), aged 5;4–9;11 years (mean: 6;7);

(ii) 10 monolingual children diagnosed with SLI (2 girls, 8 boys), aged 5;3–9;3 years (mean: 6;3);

(iii) 4 bilingual children with SLI (1 girl, 3 boys), aged 7;6–9;3 years (mean: 8;7).

Recruitment and group characteristics were the same as for Study 1.

Materials

For research purposes, Theodorou's (in progress) Cypriot Greek adaptation of the Renfrew Bus Story Test (Renfrew, 1997) was used to investigate narrative ability in three groups of children. The Bus Story Test is a screening test of verbal expression that examines story retelling with picture support. It can demonstrate difficulties with verbal expression, as well as phonological, semantic, grammatical and sequencing problems.

Procedure

The experimenter told each child the short story about the naughty red bus while the child looked through a book of pictures (but no written materials) illustrating the story. The child then retold the story, using the pictures as prompts. The narrations were recorded, transcribed, and evaluated with respect to five measures: the amount of original information included (Inf. total), the number of sentences produced (No. of sentences), word MLU, the mean sentence length of the longest five sentences (A5LS), and the number of subordinate clauses produced.

Results

Table 8.5 displays the mean scores for the five measures that were evaluated on the BST. When the bilingual SLI group was compared to the monolingual children with SLI there was no significant difference in performance on any of the subtests of the BST retell narrative: for information ($t = -2.05$, $p = 0.841$) for A5LS ($t = -0.083$, $p = 0.935$), for MLU ($t = -0.198$, $p = 0.846$), for number of sentences ($t = -0.795$, $p = 0.442$), and for number of subordinate clauses produced ($t = -0.198$, $p = 0.846$).

However, when compared to the monolingual TLD children, the bilingual group with SLI were significantly worse on A5LS ($t = 2.32$, $p = 0.036$), MLU ($t = 2.71$, $p = 0.017$), and number of subordinate clauses produced ($t = -2.709$, $p = 0.017$). In contrast, there were no significant differences between the two groups for information ($t = 1.44$, $p = 0.171$) or number of

Table 8.5 Mean scores and standard deviations (S.D.) on the Bus Story Test (BST) for participating groups

Mean	TLD (n = 12)	moSLI (n = 10)	biSLI (n = 4)
Inf. total	33.4	24.3	25.5
S.D.	9.0	9.5	11.1
MLU	4.7	2.1	2.2
S.D.	1.6	1.2	1.5
A5LS	9.3	6.6	6.7
S.D.	2.0	2.1	1.8
No. of sentences	5.3	3.85	4.24
S.D.	1.0	0.61	1.1
No. of subordinate clauses	4.7	2.3	2.3
S.D.	1.6	1.2	1.5

Key: TLD, typically language developing; moSLI, monolingual SLI; biSLI, bilingual SLI; Inf, information; MLU, mean length of utterance; A5LS, the mean sentence length of the five longest sentences.

sentences produced ($t = 1.86$, $p = 0.085$). In contrast, when the monolingual SLI group was compared to TLD peers, they performed significantly worse on all measures: information ($t = -2.31$, $p = 0.032$), A5LS ($t = -3.110$, $p = 0.006$), MLU ($t = -4.262$, $p = 0.00$), number of sentences ($t = -3.998$, $p = 0.001$), and number of subordinate clauses produced ($t = -4.262$, $p = 0.000$). We suggest caution in the interpretation of our results, given the very small number of bilingual children with SLI.

Discussion and Outlook

Cyprus has undergone major changes in population demographics and linguistic diversity over the last 20 years because of the influx of immigrants from the Balkans (former Yugoslavia, Bulgaria and Romania) and the former Soviet Union. While the global trend towards bilingual or multilingual populations is reflected in the specific sociolinguistic situation on the island of Cyprus, a pronounced shift in the kind of children requiring school-based speech language therapy services has surfaced. In the past, speech language therapy was provided exclusively to Greek Cypriot children in the standard language, Greek, but with the influx of bilingual children on SLTs' waiting lists, this has become a (new) major area of concern for two reasons. First, policy makers (such as the Ministry of Health or the Ministry of Education and Culture) have not kept up with the demographic changes – and consequently no provision has been made so far for SLT services with bilingual children. Second, at this point in time, SLTs are ill-equipped to handle this change in their core practice.

Our discussion will tie together three key topics highlighted in this chapter with regards to: (i) the relevance of our research results in discriminating bilingual children with SLI from non-impaired children; (ii) the implications for researchers in similar situations around the world, that is, where tools to diagnose SLI are currently unavailable or underdeveloped; and (iii) directions for the future.

The identification of SLI in bilingual children

The number of children who are both language impaired and speakers–hearers of two (or more) languages is growing. This is evident in rising numbers of bilingual children referred for school-based speech language pathology services in Cyprus. In contrast, prevalence measures of how common SLI is in bi- and/or multilingual children are absent. With numerical evidence lacking, we currently assume that SLI affects monolingual and bilingual children in similar numbers.

Yet, the importance of research identifying the incidence of SLI for bilingual children should not be underestimated and is something countries must strive for. Without this knowledge base, key issues important to parents, health and education professionals, policy makers and researchers involved with bilingualism will remain areas of serious contention.

Also, through our research we are collaborating closely with interpreters of different languages (unknown by us, such as Bulgarian or Romanian). Specifically, we train our interpreters on the protocol used in assessing and working with children with SLI. Our results will be made available to the relevant ministries for the provision of services and the development of policies. Furthermore, the research findings can be used by SLTs for appropriate management of bilingual children with SLI, to provide counseling to parents, to liaise with preschool teachers and to disseminate up-to-date information based on empirical research.

Moreover, the information obtained from the questionnaire sent out to SLTs (see introduction) will enable us to identify the challenges SLTs are facing, as well as their needs, and assist us in developing tools for the reliable identification of children who require clinical services. This questionnaire is relatively easy to adapt to other languages, and researchers from different countries can include language or cultural-specific issues.

Needless to say, the discovery of clinical markers for SLI in children (none identified for Cypriot Greek so far) can assist in the accurate identification of children with this disorder, and in a description of the disorder' phenotype. One challenge to this type of research is the fact that language vary in the most salient symptoms of SLI. We know now from research conducted so far that Cypriot Greek-speaking children with SLI differ from their English- and Standard Modern Greek-speaking counterparts. However, the best major characteristics that differentiate these children from their TLD compatriots remain open to investigation.

The research we have presented above revealed that in domains of language such as the lexicon and on tasks like a narrative retell, bilingual children with SLI do *not* perform that differently from their monolingual peers with SLI. In fact, the performance of bilingual children with SLI on the retrieval of verbs and nouns was comparable to that of younger, language-matched typically developing bilingual controls. In the same way, the number of sentences produced in narratives was similar to that of a monolingual TLD control group and significantly better than monolingual, but bilectal, peers with SLI.

Both findings can be used as evidence (a) in support of including bilingual children with SLI in the delayed (rather than deviant) hypothesis for SLI (Rice, 2003), and (b) that a second language does not 'worsen' the language impairment (Paradis, 2010). It is possible that, as children with SLI get older, they produce more language, as evidenced by the findings reported above regarding narratives.

Finally, the crucial question of how SLI is defined for bilingual children remains unresolved. On the European level, there is no consensus on a definition across the 27 EU member states (Cyprus included). For our current research purposes, we adopt inclusionary criteria such as the following:

- adequate hearing;
- normal non-verbal intelligence;
- normal physical development;
- no emotional/behavioral problems;
- no gross motor difficulties;
- no severe speech/articulation difficulties.

The development of linguistic measures in languages for which materials are currently unavailable in Cyprus is a major objective for targeted research, for the identification of and therapeutic measures for SLI in bi- and multilingual populations. The effort currently afforded within COST Action IS0804 (2009–2013) is a big step. Sources of bilingual language history questionnaires made available to researchers worldwide are a prerequisite for working with bilingual populations (and some can already be downloaded from the Action's website), and these are useful for determining language use, language dominance and other relevant variables in bilingual children.

Moreover, researchers need to become linguistically informed of the typical acquisition trajectories of the languages under investigation in their country before embarking on investigations or developing tools. A following step would be to develop from scratch a screening tool for any given language with language-specific areas identified as 'at-risk' markers for language impairment, similar to what we have designed as the CGLST. Potential candidates include non-word repetition, sentence recall and verb morphology (Archibald & Joanisse, 2009; see also Letts, this volume, and Chiat *et al.*, 2013). The aim is to identify children requiring further assessment.

In this sense, bilingual SLI provides the ideal opportunity for a truly multidisciplinary approach to the understanding of the disorder. The development of assessment or diagnostic tools for SLI requires the sincere collaboration between language experts (such as theoretical linguists, psycholinguists and cognitive psychologists) and SLTs.

Future directions

There is an obvious need for further research into the usefulness of the tools described above, mainly in identifying sensitivity and specificity values (Theodorou, in progress). A first objective is to design and implement a valid 'tool box', that is, provide school-based SLTs with reliable measures for the assessment of SLI. This is of overriding importance for clinical practice to avoid both under- and over-identification of SLI in bilingual populations.

A second objective is to assemble an internet portal on SLI in Cyprus, to provide users with information regarding the familial history of SLI and environmental factors for Cyprus in four languages: Greek, English, Russian and Bulgarian. Any resources will be made available upon request to parents, teachers and SLTs alike, and it will also include a section for pupils and adolescents. For academic purposes, bilingual databases will be established for use by researchers.

It is also an expressed aim of our research group, the Cyprus Acquisition Team, to work towards the development of a proper SLI laboratory in Nicosia (as was done for the UK at University College London, for example). The benefits of an SLI Lab are, among others, service provision to policy makers (more SLTs are needed) and educational seminars for early intervention professionals regarding language deficits in preschoolers (on a regular basis), including teachers and pediatricians.

Finally, we are strongly advocating the appointment of a Communication Champion (Kambanaros & Grohmann, 2011), similar to what was recommended in the 2008 Bercow review in the UK (Bercow, 2008). The role of such an individual is to work across government, delivery partners and other stakeholders in order to co-ordinate and build on initiatives to improve services for children and young people with speech, language and communication needs. We believe it is obvious that any country would benefit from such an institutionalization but, as we hope to have shown, Cyprus is a special case: it is a small country with a relatively low, yet culturally and linguistically very diverse population.

To conclude, addressing the needs of bilingual children and young people with SLI *must* achieve high political prominence in Cyprus. SLTs, parents, afflicted individuals and policy makers must collaborate and agree on a common approach to addressing the needs of communication-impaired citizens in our community. The current situation in Cyprus reflects scientific and conceptual challenges concerning the nature of these children's problems and a lack of collaborative practice between all interested parties. To achieve a systemic change across all responsible agencies and authorities (ministries) is likely to require a major government initiative.

References

Archibald, L.M.D. and Joanisse, M.F. (2009) On the sensitivity and specificity of nonword repetition and sentence recall to language and memory impairments in children. *Journal of Speech, Language and Hearing Research* 42, 899–914.

Arvaniti, A. (2006) Erasure as a means of maintaining diglossia in Cyprus. *San Diego Linguistic Papers* 2, 25–38.

Bedore, L.M. and Peña, E.D. (2008) Assessment of bilingual children for identification of language impairment: Current findings and implications for practice. *International Journal of Bilingual Education and Bilingualism* 11, 1–29.

Bercow, J. (2008) *The Bercow Report: A Review of Services for Children and Young People (0–19) with Speech, Language and Communication Needs*. Nottingham: Department for Children, Schools and Families (DCSF).

Bishop, D.V.M. (2003) *The Test for Reception of Grammar* (2nd edn). London: Pearson Assessment.

Boehm, E.A. (2000) *Boehm Test of Basic Concepts (Boehm-3)*. San Antonio, TX: Pearson.

Carrow-Woolfolk, E. (1999) *Test of Auditory Comprehension of Language* (3rd edn). Austin, TX: Pro-Ed.

Chiat, S., Armon-Lotem, S., Marinis, T., Polišenská, K., Roy, P. and Seeff-Gabriel, B. (2013) Assessment of language abilities in sequential bilingual children: The potential of sentence imitation tasks. In V.C.M. Gathercole (ed.) *Issues in the Assessment of Bilinguals* (pp. 56–89). Bristol: Multilingual Matters.

COST Action A33 (2006–2010) *Cross-Linguistically Robust Stages of Children's Linguistic Performance with Applications to the Diagnosis of SLI*. Research Network financed by the COST Office, Brussels. http://www.zas.gwz-berlin.de/cost.html?&L=0.

COST Action IS0804 (2009–2013) *Language Impairment in a Multilingual Society: Linguistic Patterns and the Road to Assessment*. Research Network financed by the COST Office, Brussels. http://www.bi-sli.org.

European Social Survey (2010) *Round 5 Source Showcards*. London: City University London, Centre for Comparative Social Surveys.

Fenson, L., Dale, P., Reznik, S., Bates, E., Thal, D. and Pethick, S. (1994) Variability in early communicative development. *Monographs of the Society for Research in Child Development* 59 (5).

Gagarina, N., Klassert, A. and Topaj, N. (2010) Russian language proficiency test for multilingual children. *ZAS Papers in Linguistics* 54. Berlin: ZAS.

Gillam, R.B. and Pearson, N. (2004) *Test of Narrative Language*. Austin, TX: Pro-Ed.

Goldman, R. and Fristoe, M. (2000) *Goldman–Fristoe Test of Articulation* (2nd edn). San Antonio, TX: Pearson.

Grohmann, K.K. and Leivada, E. (2012) Interface ingredients of dialect design: Bi-*x*, sociosyntax of development, and the grammar of Cypriot Greek. In A.M. Di Sciullo (ed.) *Towards a Biolinguistic Understanding of Grammar: Essays on the Interfaces* (pp. 239–262). Amsterdam: John Benjamins.

Hatzigeorgiou, N., Gavrilidou, M., Piperidis, S. *et al.* (2000) Design and implementation of the online ILSP corpus. *Proceedings of the Second International Conference of Language Resources and Evaluation (LREC)* 3, 1737–1740.

Justice, L.M., Bowles, R.P., Kaderavek, J.N., Ukrainetz, T.A., Eisenberg, S.L. and Gillam, R.B. (2006) The index of narrative microstructure: A clinical tool for analyzing school-age children's narrative performances. *American Journal of Speech and Language Pathology* 15, 155–191.

Kambanaros, M. (2003) Verb and noun processing in late bilingual individuals with anomic aphasia. PhD thesis, Flinders University, Adelaide.

Kambanaros, M. and Grohmann, K.K. (2010) Patterns of object and action naming in Cypriot Greek children with SLI and WFDs. In K. Franich, L. Keil, K. Iserman and J. Chandlee (eds) *Proceedings of the 34th Boston University Child Language Development – Supplement.* http://www.bu.edu/bucld/proceedings/supplement/vol34

Kambanaros, M. and Grohmann, K.K. (2011) From boys to men: How do women communication specialists fit in? In M. Koutselini and S. Agathangelou (eds) *Proceedings of the International Conference Mapping the Gender Equality: Research and Practices, 22–23 October 2010,* University of Cyprus. http://www.ucy.ac.cy/goto/unesco/en-US/publications.aspx.

Kambanaros, M., Grohmann, K.K. and Michaelides, M. (2013a) Lexical retrieval for nouns and verbs in typically developing bilectal children. *First Language.* DOI: 10.1177/0142723713479435.

Kambanaros, M., Grohmann, K.K., Michaelides, M. and Theodorou, E. (2013b) On the nature of verb–noun dissociations in bilectal SLI: A psycholinguistic perspective from Greek. *Bilingualism: Language and Cognition.* DOI: 10.1017/S1366728913000035.

Kambanaros, M., Grohmann, K.K. and Theodorou, E. (2010) Action and object naming in mono- and bilingual children with specific language impairment. In A. Botinis (ed.) *Proceedings of ISCA Tutorial and Research Workshop on Experimental Linguistics 2010, 25–27 August, Athens, Greece* (pp. 73–76). Athens: ISCA and the University of Athens.

Kambanaros, M. and Karpava, S. (2012) Comparing bilingual to monolingual children on expressive–receptive language measures. Poster presented at the Conference on Bilingual and Multilingual Interaction, 30 March–1 April, Bangor University.

Kohnert, K. (2010) Bilingual children with primary language impairment: Issues, evidence and implications for clinical actions. *Journal of Communication Disorders* 43, 456–473.

Lahey, M. and Edwards, J. (1996) Why do children with specific language impairment name pictures more slowly than peers? *Journal of Speech and Hearing Research* 30, 1081–1097.

Lahey, M. and Edwards, J. (1999) Naming errors of children with specific language impairment. *Journal of Speech Language and Hearing Research* 42, 195–205.

Li, P., Sepanski, S. and Zhao, X. (2006) Language history questionnaire: A web-based interface for bilingual research. *Behavior Research Methods* 38, 202–210.

Lyons, R., Byrne, M., Corry, T., Lalor, L., Ruane, H., Shanahan, R. and McGinty, C. (2008) An examination of how speech and language therapists assess and diagnose children with specific language impairment in Ireland. *International Journal of Speech-Language Pathology* 10, 425–437.

Miozzo, M., Costa, A., Hernandez, M. and Rapp, B. (2010) Lexical processing in the bilingual brain: Evidence from grammatical/morphological deficits. *Aphasiology* 24, 262–287.

Newton, B. (1972) *Cypriot Greek: Its Phonology and Inflections.* The Hague: Mouton.

Panhellenic Association of Logopedists (1995) *Assessment of Phonetic and Phonological Development.* Athens: PAL.

Paradis, J. (2010) Response to commentaries on the interface between bilingual development and specific language impairment. *Applied Psycholinguistics* 31, 119–136.

Paradis, J., Emmerzael, K. and Sorenson Duncan, T. (2010) Assessment of English language learners: Using parent report on first language development. *Journal of Communication Disorders* 43, 474–497.

Paraskevopoulos, J., Kalantzi-Azizi, A. and Gianitsas, N. (1999) *'Athina' Test for Diagnosis of Learning Disabilities* [in Greek]. Athens: Ellinika Grammata.

Peña, E.D. and Bedore, L. (2009) Bilingualism in child language disorders. In R.G. Schwartz (ed.) *Handbook of Child Language Disorders* (pp. 281–307). New York: Psychology Press.

Petinou, K. and Okalidou, A. (2006) Speech patterns in Cypriot Greek late talkers. *Applied Psycholinguistics* 27, 335–353.

Petinou, K. and Terzi, A. (2002) Clitic misplacement among normally developing children and children with specific language impairment and the status of Infl heads. *Language Acquisition* 10, 1–28.

Raven, J., Raven, J.C. and Court, J.H. (2000) *Manual for Raven's Progressive Matrices and Vocabulary Scales.* San Antonio, TX: Harcourt Assessment.

Renfrew, C. (1997) *The Renfrew Language Scales – Bus Story Test: A Test of Narrative Speech/Word Finding Vocabulary Test/Action Picture Test* (4th edn). Milton Keynes: Speechmark.

Rice, M.L. (2003) A unified model of specific and general language delay: Grammatical tense as a clinical marker of unexpected variation. In Y. Levy and J. Schaeffer (eds) *Language Competence across Populations: Toward a Definition of Specific Language Impairment* (pp. 63–94). Mahwah, NJ: Lawrence Erlbaum.

Rowe, C. and Grohmann, K.K. (2012) Testing the state of diglossia in Cyprus: Cypriots, binationals, and diglossic shift. Ms., University of Cyprus.

Semel, E. and Wiig, E. (1980) *Clinical Evaluation of Language Function (CELF).* Columbus, OH: Merrill.

Sheng, L. and McGregor, K.K. (2010) Object and action naming in children with specific language impairment. *Journal of Speech, Language, and Hearing Research* 53, 1704–1719.

Simos, P.G., Kasselimis, D. and Mouzaki, A. (2011) Age, gender, and education effects on vocabulary measures in Greek. *Aphasiology* 25, 475–491.

Skarakis-Doyle, E., Campbell, W. and Dempsey, L. (2009) Identification of children with language impairment: Investigating the classification accuracy of the MacArthur–Bates Communicative Development Inventories, Level III. *American Journal of Speech-Language Pathology* 18, 277–288.

Spanoudis, G., Natsopoulos, D. and Panayiotou, G. (2007) Mental verbs and pragmatic language difficulties. *International Journal of Language and Communication Disorders* 42, 487–504.

Stavrakaki, S. and Tsimpli, I.M. (2000) Diagnostic Verbal IQ Test for Greek preschool and school age children: Standardization, statistical analysis, psychometric properties [in Greek]. In *Proceedings of the 8th Conference on Speech Therapy* (pp. 95–106). Athens: Ellinika Grammata.

Theodorou, E. and Grohmann, K.K. (2010) Narratives in Cypriot Greek mono- and bilingual children with SLI. In A. Botinis (ed.) *Proceedings of ISCA Tutorial and Research Workshop on Experimental Linguistics 2010, 25–27 August, Athens, Greece* (pp. 185–188). Athens: ISCA and the University of Athens.

Thordardottir, E. (2010) Towards evidence-based practice in language intervention for bilingual children. *Journal of Communication Disorders* 43, 523–537.

Tomblin, J.B., Records, N., Buckwalter, P., Zhang, X., Smith, E. and O'Brien, M. (1997) Prevalence of specific language impairment in kindergarten children. *Journal of Speech, Language, and Hearing Research* 40, 1245–1260.

van der Lely, H.K.J. (1996) *The Test of Active and Passive Sentences (TAPS).* London: Centre for Developmental Language Disorders and Cognitive Neuroscience.

van der Lely, H.K.J. (1999) *Verb Agreement and Tense Test (VATT)*. London: Centre for Developmental Language Disorders and Cognitive Neuroscience.

Vogindroukas, I. and Grigoriadou, E. (2009) *The Test of Receptive and Expressive Language Abilities* [in Greek]. Chania: Glafki.

Vogindroukas, I., Protopappas, A. and Sideris, G. (2009) *Expressive Vocabulary Test [in Greek]*. Chania: Glafki.

Vogindroukas, I., Protopappas, A. and Stavrakaki, S. (2010) *The Greek Version of the Action Picture Test (Renfrew 1997) [in Greek]*. Chania: Glafki.

Zimmermann, I.L., Steiner, V.G. and Pond, R.E. (2002) *Preschool Language Scale* (4th edn). San Antonio, TX: Psychological Corporation.

9 Sociolinguistic Influences on the Linguistic Achievement of Bilinguals: Issues for the Assessment of Minority Language Competence

Enlli Môn Thomas, Virginia C. Mueller Gathercole and Emma K. Hughes

Developing appropriate tests for the assessment of bilinguals has received heightened attention in recent years, with testing in both languages – and on tests normed on bilingual samples – recommended as the ideal. In contexts of minority language learning, where the opportunity to hear and use the minority language can be limited, clear differences in terms of linguistic abilities are often found across different types of speakers, rendering distinct norms based on home language background an essential component of any test. This chapter examines the role of sociolinguistic factors in influencing teenagers' performance on tests of minority language competence (Welsh). It describes the process of developing standard norms for a receptive vocabulary task that include a community dominance norm in addition to a home language norm, and discusses the potential for the inclusion of detailed sociolinguistic information as part of the assessment process.

Introduction

One major concern facing educators, speech and language therapists (SLTs) and health professionals today has to do with knowing how best to serve the bilingual and multilingual children and/or adults under their care.

Bicultural and multicultural classrooms and caseloads are fast becoming the norm, and bilingualism and multilingualism a challenge to the service provider. While the academic community has continued to document critical differences between monolingual and bilingual speakers – including differences in terms of language exposure, linguistic competence and language use – the application of this knowledge in the applied setting, and to language assessment procedures in particular, has been slow. While SLTs, teachers and health professionals are often aware of these fundamental differences, they are, nonetheless, limited in the way in which they can implement their knowledge in practice and are unaware of how best to tackle some of the issues at hand. The focus of this chapter will be on speakers of a minority language in a bilingual community. The discussion will, however, be of relevance to multilingual communities and speakers also. The chapter examines some of the key factors influencing our ability to assess the linguistic achievements of bilinguals learning a minority language, with a focus on specific issues relating to the assessment of teenagers growing up in Wales.

The chapter begins with a description of the linguistic context of Wales and the nature of Welsh–English bilinguals, followed by a discussion of the problems in determining speakers' proficiency in Welsh. It then presents some recent data on teenagers' receptive vocabulary scores in Welsh, and outlines some of the critical factors – including sociolinguistic issues – that are likely to affect performance on such tasks. The chapter concludes with a discussion of the implications of the issues raised for the assessment of bilinguals and for the appropriate interpretation of assessment scores.

The linguistic context of Wales

Cymraeg (Welsh) is one of three languages that form the Brythonic branch of the Celtic family of languages (Davies, 1993). It is currently spoken by almost 600,000 speakers, approximately 21% of the population of Wales (Jones, 2012). The remaining 79% of the population are mainly English-speaking with little or no knowledge of Welsh. All L1 Welsh speakers (excluding some infants) are developing bilingually with English as their 'other' language, either as an additional first language (De Houwer, 1990; cf. 'early bilingual') – acquired simultaneously alongside Welsh – or as a very early 'second' language – acquired some time after the development of the first. At the same time, many children who begin as L1 English speakers at home but attend Welsh-medium schools also become bilingual, sometimes with Welsh as an additional first language or, more often than not, as an early second language. The focus of this chapter will be on issues relating to the assessment of the various types of bilinguals in Wales.

Following the recent passing of the Welsh Language (Wales) Measure (Welsh Government, 2011a), Welsh now holds an official status alongside English in Wales. Regardless of this new development, however, the use of the language, in actual terms, remains variable across the country. The county of Gwynedd, for example, located in the northwest region of Wales, forms part of what constitutes 'the heartland of the Welsh language' (Lindsay, 1993: 1); it is home to the largest density of speakers (Aitchison & Carter, 1994; Crystal, 1994; H.M. Jones, 2010), totalling 88% of speakers in some regions, and is home to a well-established bilingual education policy. Children attending schools in the area are educated primarily through the medium of Welsh. Outside Gwynedd, the proportion of Welsh speakers ranges from 84% in some parts of Anglesey and 75% in parts of Carmarthenshire to a maximum of 8% in Blaenau Gwent and 9% in Cardiff (Census, 2001). Nevertheless, most counties have a proportion of schools in which Welsh is the predominant language of education – a trend that continues to grow under the influence of parental pressure groups (H. Thomas, 2010). Many children from non-Welsh-speaking backgrounds attending such schools do become fully bilingual, while others develop good competence in Welsh as an early L2.

While the bilingual education system in Wales has been heralded as a great success (Welsh Government, 2010, para. 2.2), minority language education cannot by itself guarantee successful bilingualism. The fact that children are receiving Welsh as input on a daily basis at school does not necessarily result in pupils' uptake of the language (Gathercole & Thomas, 2009; Morris, 2010; Thomas & Roberts, 2011; Thomas et al., 2012), particularly in schools where the majority of children are from homes where English is the only language spoken. We will return to these points and how they may influence assessment later in the chapter.

School language statistics[1]

In 2010/2011, 419 primary schools (30% of all primary schools in Wales; 51,244 pupils in total) were classified as Welsh-medium schools (Welsh Government, 2011b: Final Results, section 7.2). A further 86 schools (6% of all primary schools in Wales; 15,910 pupils in total) made use of Welsh for part of the curriculum and/or in the day-to-day business of the school, delivering a strong Welsh ethos as a priority. The remaining 930 schools (65% of all primary schools in Wales; 192,035 pupils in total) were predominantly English-medium, teaching Welsh as a subject (and mainly as an L2).

In the same year, 32 secondary schools (SSs) (14% of all SSs in Wales; 23,033 pupils in total) were classified as Welsh-medium schools. A further 24 SSs were classified as one of three bilingual types[2] (see section 7.4 of the Schools Census document): Type A (5 schools; 3798 pupils), in which 'at least 80% of subjects, apart from English and Welsh are taught only through the medium of Welsh to all pupils . . .'; Type B (10 schools; 7787 pupils), in which 'at least 80% of subjects (excluding English and Welsh) are taught through the medium of Welsh but also taught through the medium of English'; and Type C (9 schools; 7146 pupils), in which '50–79% of subjects (excluding Welsh and English) are taught through the medium of Welsh but are also taught through the medium of English'. A further eight schools (7104 pupils) were classified as 'English with significant Welsh', bringing the total number of schools where pupils have the opportunity to learn most (or at least a substantial part) of their curriculum through the medium of Welsh up to 56 (25% of all SSs in Wales; 41,764 pupils in total). However, the majority of SSs in Wales (158 SSs (71% of all SSs); 152,362 pupils) were classified as English-medium.

What these figures demonstrate is that all children attending main-stream schools in Wales are encouraged to learn Welsh, either as a taught subject as part of the curriculum or by receiving their education wholly or partially through the medium of Welsh. The recent obligation to learn Welsh until age 16 years at school (as outlined first in the Education Act of 1988) has led to an increase in the number of Welsh speakers (and, hence, bilin-guals); over 40% of the population identified as Welsh speakers in the 2001 Census were children between the ages of 5 and 15 (Morris, 2010; Jones, 2012). While this pattern of 'revival' is a welcome development, there remains a continued concern that children (and teenagers in particular) are reluctant to use the language outside the education context (see Morris, 2010; Thomas & Roberts, 2011; Thomas et al., 2012), particularly in (but not limited to) the more Anglicized areas of Wales. If, as Eilers et al. (2006: 71) suggest, 'the bottom line for successful bilingualism is whether one uses two languages consistently', this reluctance to use the language may lead to underachieve-ment in one or both of a bilinguals' languages, which may be difficult to distinguish from a clinical language disorder. We will return to this point later in this chapter.

Although fairly homogenous, then, in terms of the types of languages spoken by the children (i.e. Welsh and/or English, with some instances of children speaking (an)other language(s) at home), Welsh classrooms are mainly a mixture of simultaneous and successive bilinguals (Lewis, 2004) whose linguistic abilities reflect their patterns of exposure to, and use of, the language (see below). *All* children who are educated either wholly or partially through the medium of Welsh are bilingual to some extent, and should never be treated – or tested – as if they were the same as monolingual speakers of English (or, indeed, of Welsh). (However, Thordardottir (2011: 441) cautions that while it is imperative not to expect bilinguals to achieve monolingual norms too early, it is also important not to underestimate their abilities to do so.) The next section describes some of the problems facing educators, SLTs and health practitioners in determining a given bilingual child's proficiency in Welsh.

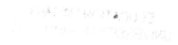

Determining linguistic abilities: The difficulties in Wales

As mentioned above, Welsh–English bilinguals are not one 'type' (cf. Grosjean, 1998; Nicoladis, 2008; Romaine, 1995; Wei, 2000). The exact nature of bilinguals' linguistic knowledge will vary from one individual to the next, depending on their linguistic experiences (Grosjean, 1998, 2000; Li, 1996). These experiences differ in many ways, including variations in amount of exposure (Oller, 2005; Oller & Eilers, 2002; Thordardottir, 2011), age of acquisition (Johnson & Newport, 1989; Mayberry, 2007), quality of exposure (Chondrogianni & Marinis, 2011; Döpke, 1988; Hulk & Cornips, 2006), and many other psychosocial variables, including parental and individual attitudes and motivation (Baker, 1992; Bartram, 2006; Cenoz, 2003; Chumak-Horbatsch, 2008; Dörnyei, 2001, 2006; Luo & Weisman, 2000; Lyon, 1996; Oliver & Purdie, 1998).

We already know from the psycholinguistic literature that the frequency with which language(s) are spoken in the child's home – and, to a lesser extent, at school – influences children's development of certain structures. In relation to lexical development, for example, the amount of exposure seems to have a direct influence on children's vocabulary knowledge, not only in the monolingual setting (e.g. Hart & Risely, 1995; Huttenlocher *et al.*, 1991) but also in the bilingual/L2 setting (e.g. Cobo-Lewis *et al.*, 2002a, 2002b; Gathercole *et al.*, 2008; Pearson *et al.*, 1993, 1997; Umbel *et al.*, 1992). Similar trends have also been found for children's acquisition of morphosyntactic constructs (Blom, 2011; Gathercole, 1986, 2002a, 2002b, 2002c; Gathercole *et al.*, 1999; Hoff *et al.*, 2012; Maratsos, 2000; Thordardottir *et al.*, 2006). Together, these studies highlight the fact that the more a child is exposed to direct linguistic input, the quicker and better their linguistic attainments in the language(s) they are hearing. In the bilingual setting this is even more crucial since no bilingual is ever able to devote 100% of his or her time to developing only one of the languages (Paradis, 2010a). As a result, bilinguals may take longer to accumulate the 'critical mass of exposure' (Gathercole, 2007b ; Marchman & Bates, 1994) that is necessary for sorting out the grammatical systems they are learning, to develop extensive vocabulary or to consolidate the meanings of words. They may therefore lag behind their monolingual peers at certain points in development (Bialystok *et al.*, 2010; Oller & Eilers, 2002).

One explanation for this 'bilingual delay' is that, for bilinguals, language learning may be domain-specific (Li, 1996), leading to a *distributed* knowledge of certain aspects of language (cf. *Complementarity Principle*; Grosjean, 1998, 2000). That is, bilinguals 'share' their languages across domains such that they may learn words and expressions for science, for example, in one language (the language of the school), words and expressions for cooking and eating in another (the language of the home), but may have words and expressions for playing and having fun in both languages. Such 'diglossic' use of languages (Ferguson, 1959) means that a bilingual's linguistic repertoire is thus distributed across their two languages, depending on the linguistic medium of their experiences (the so-called *distributed characteristic* of bilinguals; Oller, 2005). Consequently, their vocabulary stores, in either of their two languages, may be smaller than that of their monolingual peers (particularly when testing productive vocabulary; e.g. Thordardottir, 2011; Thordardottir *et al.*, 2006), which may lead to extensive borrowing, especially when using their weaker language (Genesee *et al.*, 1995; Lanvers, 2001). In time, bilinguals can develop translation equivalents and expand their vocabulary across domains, provided they have the opportunity to engage with the other language in a variety of contexts (Bahrick *et al.*, 1994; but cf. Bialystok & Luk, 2012). Similarly, purported early delays in morphosyntactic knowledge seem to 'level out' at later stages, once the child has accumulated enough experience with the language. In some cases, bilinguals may even demonstrate accelerated performance as compared to monolingual age-matched peers, whereby knowledge of a structure in language A may bolster the child's knowledge of a similar (and often more complex) structure in language B (Fabiano-Smith & Barlow, 2009; Kupisch, 2006; Paradis & Genesee, 1996). Yet, a reported lag in vocabulary and/or morphosyntactic knowledge is often misinterpreted as evidence of a language disorder, and is partially responsible for the over-representation of bilinguals – especially L2 speakers of English – in many Special Education units and schools (Paradis *et al.*, 2007, 2008; see Kambanaros & Grohmann, this volume). Also noteworthy is the fact that L2 children's patterns of linguistic development can overlap with those of children with specific language impairment (SLI) (Crago & Paradis, 2003; Letts, this volume; Paradis, 2004, 2005; although there are also certain differences – Paradis, 2010b), adding a further dimension to the problems of differential diagnosis.

In the Welsh context in particular, studies have highlighted the role of input factors (in terms of amount of exposure, at least) in children's acquisition of gender and word order (Gathercole & Thomas, 2005, 2009; Gathercole *et al.*, 2001, 2005), as well as in terms of vocabulary development (Gathercole & Thomas, 2009; Rhys & Thomas, 2012). More recent examinations are also investigating the interaction between quantity (in terms of frequency of exposure) and quality (in terms of consistency and reliability) of input in development (Thomas *et al.*, under review, for plural morphology; Lloyd-Williams & Thomas, in preparation, for the answering system). Together, these studies highlight the combinatory roles of internal and external factors in guiding children's linguistic achievements. When exposure is frequent, and the structures are used consistently, providing reliable cues to form-function mappings, the quicker, and 'fuller' the child's acquisition of complex structures in Welsh. Language measures developed for use with bilinguals need to be sensitive to such variations across different types of bilingual speakers in two ways: first, careful selection of appropriate linguistic items or structures can help discriminate meaningfully between typical and atypical linguistic behaviour; and, second, appropriate norming samples can aid in comparing a given bilingual child's performance to relevant peers.

A language assessment measure that attempts to account for the differences across various types of bilinguals in Wales is the *Prawf Geirfa Cymraeg: Fersiwn 7–11* ('Welsh Vocabulary Test') developed by Gathercole and Thomas (2007b) (see Gathercole *et al.*, 2008, 2013). This is the first ever standardized test of receptive vocabulary available in Welsh. This test was developed as a measure of receptive vocabulary knowledge and was normed on a sample of 611 children. This measure has the unique characteristic that each child receives two standardized scores, one of which places the child's performance in the context of the overall performance of children of the same age, the other of which places the child's performance relative to children of the same 'type' (those from predominantly Welsh-speaking, from mixed Welsh- and English-speaking, or from predominantly English-speaking homes) at each age/school year. An adapted version of this test for 11- to 15-year-olds has recently been completed (see Gathercole *et al.*, in preparation), which has revealed some interesting patterns that warrant further discussion. These patterns are discussed below.

Teenagers' Receptive Command of Vocabulary in Welsh

Seven hundred and sixty-seven children between the ages of 11 and 15 took part in a forced-choice receptive vocabulary test, based on the previous version developed for 7- to 11-year-olds (Gathercole & Thomas, 2007b; Gathercole *et al.*, 2008, 2013, in press). The children came from three distinct home language types: Only Welsh at Home ('OWH'), in which parents spoke only or mainly Welsh to the child; Welsh and English Homes ('WEH'), in which parents spoke both Welsh and English to the child (either in a one-parent one-language situation or with one or both parents speaking both languages to the child); and Only English Homes ('OEH'), in which parents spoke only or mostly English to the child. The number of children per home language type and by age can be seen in Table 9.1 (see Gathercole *et al.*, in press, for further information).

The version of the task developed for 11- to 15-year-olds involved 212 of the same items that appeared in the original testing pool of words for the task for the younger children, plus 30 less frequent words, making a total of 242 words to test. These words represented seven different frequency levels (as found in Ellis *et al.*'s (2001) one million-word lexical database and frequency count for Welsh written words – see Gathercole & Thomas, 2007b and Gathercole *et al.*, 2008 for a description of the various frequency levels). Of these 242 words, performance on 125 of the words was at ceiling (over

Table 9.1 Participant sample

Home language	Age					Total
	11	12	13	14	15	
OWH	47	57	48	56	52	260
WEH	35	69	45	49	41	239
OEH	31	54	54	77	52	268
Total	113	180	147	182	145	767

90% correct responses) or at baseline (under 25% correct responses); these items were eliminated from the final test. An additional three words were non-discriminatory, in that performance on these words did not differ in a significant way either by age or home language. These items were also eliminated from the final test. This yielded a total of 114 words that could be used to assess performance by individual children and across groups.

The performance of the 11- to 15-year-olds on the 114 discriminating words is presented in Figure 9.1. Analyses revealed that the general pattern was one of continual progression across ages, especially among the OWH and WEH children. (See Gathercole *et al.*, in press, for statistical analyses.) The performance of the OEH children, however, appeared more uniform across

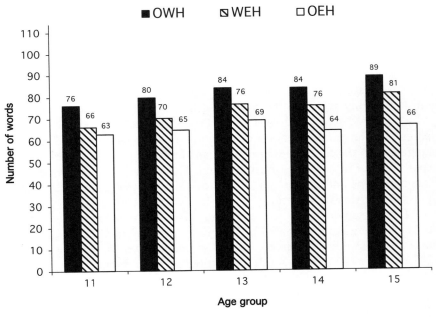

Figure 9.1 Performance on the *Prawf Geirfa Cymraeg* by home language and age

ages. This lack of continued progression during the secondary school years reflects a growing trend in Wales that features clearly in the recent Welsh-Medium Education Strategy (Welsh Government, 2010). To explore these results, we separated those children who were living in communities in which over 65% of the population were speakers of Welsh and those who were living in communities with lower percentages of Welsh speakers. Analyses again revealed that, while the performance of the OWH and WEH children in these two types of areas did not differ significantly, the performance of the OEH children differed in the two types of communities (see Figure 9.2). In those communities with the higher percentage of Welsh speakers, the OEH performance, like that of the OWH and WEH children, improved with age. However, in the communities with fewer Welsh speakers, the OEH children's performance did not improve at ages 14 and 15, and it was significantly worse than that of the OEH 14- and 15-year-olds in the more dominant Welsh communities.

These data demonstrate clearly that after age 13, if children from OEH backgrounds live in communities where less Welsh is spoken, they may fail to advance in their Welsh vocabulary knowledge. Therefore, the community in which they are growing up matters for expectations about their knowledge of Welsh vocabulary. These findings pose certain challenges when aiming to develop standardized norms for Welsh-speaking bilinguals. In this case, our

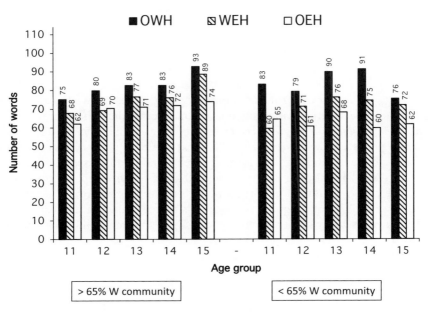

Figure 9.2 Performance on the *Prawf Geirfa Cymraeg* by home language, age and community type

solution has been as follows. First, at all ages, children receive two standardized scores, as in the 7–11 version of the *PGC* – one according to all children of their age group, and one according to their home language profile. However, at ages 14 and 15, we have divided the OEH children according to the prevalence of Welsh speakers in their communities, so that OEH children receive their second standard score not only on the basis of home language but also taking into consideration their community language (see Gathercole *et al.*, in press, for further details).

Children's attainment levels in each of their languages can thus differ dramatically in bilingual community settings, and can vary from one community to the next. The attainment appears to be influenced by a number of factors, including: (1) language dominance patterns in the community; (2) language use in peer-to-peer interactions; and (3) potential imbalance in the domains of language use. Profiling bilingual children's experiences with language along these dimensions may offer key aspects of information that can help aid with the interpretation of test results, for the reasons outlined below.

Language dominance

A number of studies have highlighted the role of language dominance, both in society and within the individual, in influencing bilingual children's linguistic attainments (Oller & Eilers, 2002; Paradis, 2010a, 2010b; Paradis *et al.*, 2008). For example, we (Gathercole & Thomas, 2009; Gathercole *et al.*, 2013) have demonstrated that children's receptive knowledge of English vocabulary becomes more similar across different home language backgrounds before children's knowledge of Welsh vocabulary does. In some studies we have seen children's abilities in English vocabulary coming together as early as age 8 years regardless of home language exposure, with performance on Welsh becoming similar much later. In other studies, the timing appears to be later, even for English. For example, Rhys and Thomas (2012) demonstrate persistent differences at age 11 across home language types for vocabulary knowledge and reading, for both Welsh and English; see also Bialystok *et al.* (2010) for similar results at age 10 for English receptive vocabulary. Gathercole *et al.* (2013), report similarly on studies revealing that children from various home language backgrounds perform alike on English vocabulary by ages 13 to 15, but at this age the OEH children still lag behind their OWH and WEH peers on Welsh vocabulary. We have argued that since English is the more pervasive language, children have the opportunity to hear and use English across many more domains than they might for Welsh. Consequently, bilingual children in Wales are more likely to experience incomplete acquisition of Welsh than they are to experience incomplete acquisition of English. In a similar vein, Paradis (2010b) has argued that the 'projected linguistic outcomes' (Paradis, 2010b: 228) of bilinguals may be influenced by the sociolinguistic dominance patterns between their two languages. Children living in areas where there are two majority languages (e.g. French and English in Canada) are likely to gain full competence in both languages, whereas children speaking a minority home language, learning the dominant societal language at school, are more likely to suffer incomplete acquisition or attrition in their L1 (Paradis, 2010b). In the Welsh context, our studies demonstrate that children learning the dominant societal language at home (English) and the minority status language at school (Welsh) continue to progress at the same level as (near-) monolingual English speakers in English, but their ultimate attainment in Welsh may be more uncertain. Children from minority language status homes (Welsh) learning the same minority language at school may progress well in both languages.

Influence of peer-to-peer interactions

A number of studies have highlighted the role of peers in shaping children's linguistic behaviours (Gathercole, 2007a; Gathercole & Thomas, 2007a; Thomas, 2007; Vihman, 1998). The extent to which children use each language in various contexts – including beyond the educational setting – varies from one individual to the next and may have direct consequences on linguistic behaviour. In the French–English context in Canada, for example, 'students gain fluency and literacy in French at no apparent cost to their English academic skills' (Cummins, 1998: 34), a pattern that has been found for diverse immersion programmes (e.g. Johnstone, 2002; Ramírez et al., 1991), even late immersion (Genesee, 1983). However, although L2 French children's mastery of English and their receptive skills in French are reported to be native-like from an early age, their productive skills in French tend to lag behind those of native L1 speakers, even at Grade 6 (Harley et al., 1991; Lapkin et al., 1990; see also Thordardottir, 2011). This may be influenced by children's reluctance to use their L2 in social contexts, particularly in peer-to-peer interactions: Genesee (1978) noted that children attending French immersion schooling in Canada tended to use English in the wider community, limiting their use of French to the school context. Similar patterns of use have also been documented for Spanish in the Miami context, with increasing use of English across elementary school (Eilers et al., 2006), and for Mexican-American teenagers in California (Hakuta & D'Andrea, 1992).

A recent study commissioned by the Welsh Language Board (2006) (also reported in Morris, 2010) looked at Welsh-speaking teenagers' social networks and investigated their use of language in interpersonal interactions. Twenty-four 13- to 17-year-olds from various home language backgrounds were recruited in each of twelve geographical areas across Wales.

The results revealed a marked decrease in the use of Welsh among older informants, particularly with friends, but also with teachers. The extent to which children from Welsh-speaking families engaged with Welsh in their social activities outside school was largely dependent on their geographical area, with as few as 2% of children from Welsh-speaking families living in Fishguard using Welsh in social networks and as many as 94% doing so in Bala. Especially children from English-speaking backgrounds and almost *all* children living in English-dominant areas largely choose to use English with their friends. For these children, engagement with spoken Welsh is limited to the classroom, and largely in interaction with the teacher. But even in regions where Welsh is the majority language and where Welsh-medium education is the norm, this preference to converse in English is also observed (Thomas & Roberts, 2011).

Domains of language use

Practice across many social domains is a key factor in the long-term maintenance of bilingualism (Escamilla, 1994: 23). Yet, bilinguals may be limited in their use of one or both of their languages in various domains, and with various individuals, possibly curbing optimal achievement in either one or the other of their languages. The extent to which children engage in informal interactions in their minority L2 (or even L1) in any (or all) of these contexts may have direct consequences for linguistic outcomes as well as for educational success. For many bilinguals in Wales, exposure to Welsh is limited to the education domain. In the Welsh Language Board study (2006; Morris, 2010), for example, children's confidence in using Welsh was reported to vary across domains, with teenagers being most confident using Welsh with known adults (56% very confident, 26% confident) and least confident with unknown contemporaries and unknown adults (26–27% very confident, 26–27% confident). Teenagers may thus avoid using Welsh with some individuals, limiting the expanse of their experience with the language. Similar findings are reported in Thomas and Roberts (2011) for primary school-aged children. Test developers may wish to consider such matters when devising their tasks: Should tests measuring the Welsh language abilities of children exposed to Welsh at school focus on the typical vocabulary and structures that abound in the more formal, academic setting? Should tests developed for L1 speakers of Welsh cover a broader range of styles (both formal and informal), reflecting their broader experience in various domains of Welsh language use?

Implications for Assessment

The upshot of the above data and issues discussed in this chapter is that, depending on the targeted goal for measuring a child's knowledge of the language (see Gathercole, 2010), at times the ideal would be to develop tests for the assessment of bilingual speakers' linguistic abilities that are normed relative to the 'type' of bilingual of concern. In the Welsh–English context, for example, at least for certain purposes, this means formulating separate norms for those learning Welsh as an L1 at home, those exposed to both Welsh and English at home from birth, and those exposed to English as their L1 at home but who are exposed to Welsh at school. However, home language norms by themselves may not always be enough. While it may be unrealistic to develop norms that control for all possible variations in bilinguals' linguistic experiences, collecting information on speakers' full linguistic profiles – including measures of language *use*, inclusive of the school/home setting and beyond – is vital in order to ensure appropriate testing and/or interpretation of results. Observed or documented differences in use across groups (by gender, by home language experiences, by linguistic make-up of the school and area) may be important to consider in the assessment process. It is in the combination of detailed psychometric testing (normed for bilinguals) and descriptive measures of language ability and use that we may best be able to serve the needs of bilingual speakers and inform best practice for therapy and action.

Summary and Conclusions

This chapter has outlined a number of reasons why the determination of a bilingual speaker's linguistic abilities can be a challenge. As suggested by others in these volumes, a reliable measure of bilinguals' language abilities should involve testing in both languages, and using tests normed on age-matched bilingual children with similar linguistic experiences. However, obtaining such 'norms' in bilingual situations is clearly a challenge. It is at times important to consider factors that are known to influence minority speakers' use and acquisition of language – including those that go beyond the medium of linguistic exchange at home and at school – and they should then be considered in the assessment process itself. Only when thoughtful consideration is given to such factors can practitioners and educators working under conditions of minority language survival provide the best service to the bilingual and multilingual children in their care.

Acknowledgements

This work was supported in part by ESRC & WAG/HEFCW grant RES-535-30-0061, ESRC grant RES-062-23-0175, and a WAG grant on the Continued Development of Standardized Measures for the Assessment of Welsh, for which we are very grateful. We also wish to thank the schools, parents, and children who participated in the studies reported here, and Emily Roberts and Catrin Hughes for their assistance in the analysis of the data from the 11- to 15-year-old children.

Notes

(1) See, for example, B. Jones (2010), Baker (1993) and Lewis (2008) for reviews of the complexities of the multiple terms used to describe schools in Wales according to the proportion of use of Welsh in classrooms across Wales.
(2) Although a fourth type exists (Type 'Ch'), there were no schools of this type in 2010/2011.

References

Aitchison, J.W. and Carter, H. (1994) *A Geography of the Welsh Language 1961–1991*. Cardiff: University of Wales Press.
Bahrick, H.P., Hall, L.K., Goggin, J.P., Bahrick, L.E. and Berger, S.A. (1994) Fifty years of language maintenance and language dominance in bilingual Hispanic immigrants. *Journal of Experimental Psychology* 123 (3), 264–283.
Baker, C.R. (1992) *Attitudes and Language*. Clevedon: Multilingual Matters.
Baker, C.R. (1993) Bilingual education in Wales. In H. Baetens Beardsmore (ed.) *European Models of Bilingual Education* (pp. 7–29). Clevedon: Multilingual Matters.
Bartram, B. (2006) Attitudes to language learning: A comparative study of peer group influences. *Language Learning Journal* 33, 47–52.
Bialystok, E. and Luk, G. (2012) Receptive vocabulary differences in monolingual and bilingual adults. *Bilingualism: Language and Cognition* 15 (2), 397–401.
Bialystok, E., Luk, G., Peets, K.F. and Yang, S. (2010) Receptive vocabulary differences in monolingual and bilingual children. *Bilingualism: Language and Cognition* 13 (4), 525–531.
Blom, E. (2011) Effects of input on the early grammatical development of bilingual children. *International Journal of Bilingualism* 14, 422–446.
Cenoz, J. (2003) The influence of age on the acquisition of English: General proficiency, attitudes and code mixing. In M. Garcia Mayo and M. Garcia Lecumberri (eds) *Age and the Acquisition of English as a Foreign Language* (pp. 77–93). Clevedon: Multilingual Matters.
Census (2001) *Percentage of Population Age 3 and Over Welsh Speaking According to 2001 Census of Population*. 2001 Census. Crown copyright.
Chondrogianni, V. and Marinis, T. (2011) Differential effects of internal and external factors on the development of vocabulary, tense morphology and morpho-syntax in successive bilingual children. *Linguistic Approaches to Bilingualism* 1 (3), 318–345; doi: 10.1075/lab.1.3.05cho.
Chumak-Horbatsch, R. (2008) Early bilingualism: Children of immigrants in an English-language childcare centre. *Psychology of Language and Communication* 12 (1), 3–27.
Cobo-Lewis, A., Pearson, B., Eilers, R. and Umbel, V. (2002a) Effects of bilingualism and bilingual education on oral and written English skills: A multifactor study of standardized test outcomes. In D.K. Oller and R.E. Eilers (eds) *Language and Literacy in Bilingual Children* (pp. 64–97). Clevedon: Multilingual Matters.
Cobo-Lewis, A., Pearson, B., Eilers, R. and Umbel, V. (2002b) Effects of bilingualism and bilingual education on oral and written Spanish skills: A multifactor study of standardized test outcomes. In D.K. Oller and R.E. Eilers (eds) *Language and Literacy in Bilingual Children* (pp. 98–117). Clevedon: Multilingual Matters.
Crago, M. and Pradis, J. (2003) Two of a kind? Commonalities and variation in language and language learners. In Y. Levy and J. Schaeffer (eds) *Language Competence Across Populations: Towards a Definition of Specific Language Impairment* (pp. 97–110). Mahwah, NJ: Erlbaum.
Crystal, D. (1994) *An Encyclopaedic Dictionary of Language and Languages*. Harmondsworth: Penguin Books.

Sociolinguistic Influences on the Linguistic Achievement of Bilinguals 189

Cummins, J. (1998) Immersion education for the millennium: What have we learned from 30 years of research on second language immersion? In M.R. Childs and R.M. Bostwick (eds) *Learning Through Two Languages: Research and Practice. Second Katoh Gakuen International Symposium on Immersion and Bilingual Education* (pp. 34–47). Shizuoka: Katoh Gakuen.

Davies, J. (1993) *The Welsh Language*. Cardiff: University of Wales Press.

De Houwer, A. (1990) *The Acquisition of Two Languages from Birth: A Case Study*. Cambridge: Cambridge University Press.

Döpke, S. (1988) The role of parental teaching techniques in bilingual German–English families. *International Journal of the Sociology of Language* 72, 101–112.

Dörnyei, Z. (2001) *Teaching and Researching Motivation*. Harlow: Pearson Education.

Dörnyei, Z. (2006) Individual differences in second language acquisition. *AILA Review* 19, 42–68.

Eilers, R.E., Pearson, B.Z. and Cobol-Lewis, A. (2006) Social factors in bilingual development: The Miami experience. In P. McCardle and E. Hoff (eds) *Childhood Bilingualism: Research on Infancy Through School Age* (pp. 68–90). Clevedon: Multilingual Matters.

Ellis, N.C., O'Dochartaigh, C., Hicks, W., Morgan, M. and Laporte, N. (2001) *CronfaElectroneg o Gymraeg/A 1 Million Word Lexical Database and Frequency Count for Welsh*. Bangor: School of Psychology, University of Wales Bangor. http://www.bangor.ac.uk/canolfanbedwyr/ceg.php.en

Escamilla, K. (1994) The sociolinguistic environment of a bilingual school: A case study introduction. *Bilingual Research Journal* 18 (1/2), 22–47.

Fabiano-Smith, L. and Barlow, J.A. (2009) Interaction in bilingual phonological acquisition: Evidence from phonetic inventories. *International Journal of Bilingual Education and Bilingualism*, 31 (1), 1–17.

Ferguson, C.A. (1959) Diglossia. *Word* 15, 324–340.

Gathercole, V.C.M. (1986) Evaluating competing linguistic theories with child language data: The case of the mass-count distinction. *Linguistics and Philosophy* 9, 151–190.

Gathercole, V.C.M. (2002a) Command of the mass/count distinction in bilingual and monolingual children: An English morphosyntactic distinction. In D.K. Oller and R.E. Eilers (eds) *Language and Literacy in Bilingual Children* (pp. 175–206). Clevedon: Multilingual Matters.

Gathercole, V.C.M. (2002b) Grammatical gender in bilingual and monolingual children: A Spanish morphosyntactic distinction. In D.K. Oller and R.E. Eilers (eds) *Language and Literacy in Bilingual Children* (pp. 207–219). Clevedon: Multilingual Matters.

Gathercole, V.C.M. (2002c) Monolingual and bilingual acquisition: Learning different treatments of *that*-trace phenomena in English and Spanish. In D.K. Oller and R.E. Eilers (eds) *Language and Literacy in Bilingual Children* (pp. 220–254). Clevedon: Multilingual Matters.

Gathercole, V.C.M. (2007a) Concerted influences on language transmission: Summary and discussion. In V.C. Gathercole (ed.) *Language Transmission in Bilingual Families in Wales*. Cardiff: Welsh Language Board.

Gathercole, V.C.M. (2007b) Miami and North Wales, so far and yet so near: Constructivist account of morpho-syntactic development in bilingual children. *International Journal of Bilingual Education and Bilingualism* 10 (3), 224–247.

Gathercole, V.C.M. (2010) Bilingual children: Language and assessment issues for educators. In K. Littleton, C. Wood and J. Kleine Staarman (eds) *Handbook of Psychology in Education* (pp. 713–748). Bingley: Emerald Group.

Gathercole, V.C.M., Laporte, N.I. and Thomas, E.M. (2005) Differentiation, carry-over, and the distributed characteristic in bilinguals: Structural 'mixing' of the two languages? In J. Cohen, K. McAlister, K. Rolstad and J. MacSwan (eds) *ISB4: Proceedings of the 4th International Symposium on Bilingualism* (pp. 838–851). Somerville, MA: Cascadilla Press.

Gathercole, V.C.M., Sebastián, E. and Soto, P. (1999) The early acquisition of Spanish verbal morphology: Across-the-board or piecemeal knowledge? *International Journal of Bilingualism* 3 (2/3), 133–182.

Gathercole, V.C.M. and Thomas, E.M. (2005) Minority language survival: Input factors influencing the acquisition of Welsh. In J. Cohen, K.T. McAlister, K. Rolstad and J. MacSwan (eds) *Proceedings of the 4th International Symposium on Bilingualism* (pp. 852–874). Somerville, MA: Cascadilla Press.

Gathercole, V.C.M. and Thomas, E.M. (2007a) Factors contributing to language transmission in bilingual families: The core study – adult interviews. In V.C. Gathercole (ed.) *Language Transmission in Bilingual Families in Wales*. Cardiff: Welsh Language Board.

Gathercole, V.C.M. and Thomas, E.M. (2007b) *Prawf Geirfa Cymraeg: Fersiwn 7–11*. Bangor: School of Psychology, Bangor University. http://www.pgc.bangor.ac.uk

Gathercole, V.C.M. and Thomas, E.M. (2009) Bilingual first-language development: Dominant language takeover, threatened minority language take-up. *Bilingualism: Language and Cognition* 12 (2), 213–237.

Gathercole, V.C.M., Thomas, E.M. and Hughes, E.K. (2008) Designing a normed receptive vocabulary test for bilingual populations: A model from Welsh. *International Journal of Bilingual Education and Bilingualism* 11 (6), 678–720.

Gathercole, V.C.M., Thomas, E.M., Hughes, E.K., Roberts, E.J. and Hughes, C. (in press) *Prawf Geirfa Cymraeg: Fersiwn 11–15*. Bangor: School of Psychology, Bangor University.

Gathercole, V.C.M., Thomas, E.M. and Laporte, N.I. (2001) The acquisition of grammatical gender in Welsh. *Journal of Celtic Language Learning* 6, 53–87.

Gathercole, V.C.M., Thomas, E.M., Roberts, E., Hughes, C. and Hughes, E.K. (2013) Why assessment needs to take exposure into account: Vocabulary and grammatical abilities in bilingual children. In V.C.M. Gathercole (ed.) *Issues in the Assessment of Bilinguals* (pp. 20–55). Bristol: Multilingual Matters.

Genesee, F. (1978) Scholastic effects of French immersion: An overview after ten years. *Interchange* 9 (4), 20–28.

Genesee, F. (1983) Bilingual education of minority-language children: The immersion experiments in review. *Applied Psycholinguistics* 4 (1), 1–46.

Genesee, F., Nicoladis, E. and Paradis, J. (1995) Language differentiation in early bilingual development. *Journal of Child Language* 22, 611–631.

Grosjean, F. (1998) Studying bilinguals: Methodological and conceptual issues. *Bilingualism: Language and Cognition* 1, 131–149.

Grosjean, F. (2000) *Life with Two Languages: An Introduction to Bilingualism*. Cambridge, MA: Harvard University Press.

Hakuta, K. and D'Andrea, D. (1992) Some properties of bilingual maintenance and loss in Mexican background high-school students. *Applied Linguistics* 13 (1), 72–99.

Harley, B., Allen, P., Cummins, J. and Swain, M. (1991) *The Development of Second Language Proficiency*. Cambridge: Cambridge University Press.

Hart, B. and Risely, T.R. (1995) *Meaningful Differences in the Everyday Experience of Young American Children*. Baltimore, MD: Brookes Publishing.

Hoff, E., Core, C., Place, S., Rumiche, R., Señor, M. and Parra, M. (2012) Dual language exposure and early bilingual development. *Journal of Child Language* 39 (1), 1–27.

Hulk, A.J. and Cornips, L. (2006) The acquisition of definite determiners in child L2 Dutch: Problems with neuter gender nouns. In S. Unsworth, T. Parodi, A. Sorace and M. Young-Scholten (eds) *Paths of Development in L1 and L2 Acquisition* (pp. 107–134). Amsterdam: John Benjamins.

Huttenlocher, J., Haight, W., Bryk, M., Seltzer, M. and Lyons, T. (1991) Early vocabulary growth: Relation to language input and gender. *Developmental Psychology* 27, 236–248.

Johnson, J.S. and Newport, E.L. (1989) Critical period effects in second language learning: The influence of maturational state on the acquisition of English as a second language. *Cognitive Psychology* 21, 60–99.

Johnstone, R. (2002) *Immersion in a Second or Additional Language at School: A Review of the International Research*. Stirling: Scottish CiLT.

Jones, B. (2010) Amrywaieth 'Caleidosgopic': adysg ddwyieithog yng Nghymru heddiw. *Gwerddon* 5. http://www.gwerddon.org/cy/rhifynnau/rhifynnaugwerddon/teitl-3528-cy.aspx

Jones, H.M. (2010) Welsh speakers: Age profile and out-migration. In D. Morris (ed.) *Welsh in the Twenty-First Century* (pp. 118–147). Cardiff: Cardiff University Press.

Jones, H.M. (2012) *A Statistical Overview of the Welsh Language*. Cardiff: Welsh Language Board.

Kupisch, T. (2006) *The Acquisition of Determiners in Bilingual German-Italian and German-French Children*. München: Lingcom Europa.

Lanvers, U. (2001) Language alternation in infant bilinguals: A developmental approach to codeswitching. *International Journal of Bilingualism* 5, 437–464.

Lapkin, S., Swain, M. and Shapson, S. (1990) French immersion research agenda for the 90s. *Canadian Modern Language Review* 46, 638–674.

Lewis, W.G. (2004) Addysg Gynradd Gymraeg: Trochi ac Ymestyn Disgyblion/Welsh primary education: Immersing and enriching pupils. *Welsh Journal of Education* 12 (2), 48–64.

Lewis, W.G. (2008) Current challenges in bilingual education in Wales. In *Multilingualism and Minority Languages: Achievements and Challenges in Education. AILA Review* (Vol 21; pp. 69–86). Amsterdam: John Benjamins.

Li, D.C.S. (1996) *Issues in Bilingualism and Biculturalism: A Hong Kong Case Study* (Vol. 21). New York: Peter Lang.

Lindsay, C.F. (1993) Welsh and English in the city of Bangor: A study in functional differentiation. *Language in Society* 22, 1–17.

Lloyd-Williams, S.W. and Thomas, E.M. (in preparation) Factors influencing bilinguals' acquisition complex structures: The case of Welsh-English children's acquisition of the Welsh answering system.

Luo, S.H. and Weisman, R.L. (2000) Ethnic language maintenance among Chinese immigrant children in the United States. *International Journal of Intercultural Relations* 24, 307–324.

Lyon, J. (1996) *Becoming Bilingual: Language Acquisition in a Bilingual Community*. Clevedon: Multilingual Matters.

Maratsos, M. (2000) More overregularizations after all. *Journal of Child Language* 28, 32–54.

Marchman, V.A. and Bates, E. (1994) Continuity in lexical and morphological development: A test of the critical mass hypothesis. *Journal of Child Language* 21, 339–366.

Mayberry, R.I. (2007) When timing is everything: Age of first-language acquisition effects in second-language learning. *Applied Psycholinguistics* 28, 537–549

Morris, D. (2010) Young people and their use of the Welsh language. In D. Morris (ed.) *Welsh in the Twenty-First Century* (pp. 80–98). Cardiff: Cardiff University Press.

Nicoladis, E. (2008) Bilingualism and language cognitive development. In J. Altarriba and R.R. Heredia (eds) *An Introduction to Bilingualism: Principles and Processes* (pp. 167–184). Mahwah, NJ: Lawrence Erlbaum.

Oliver, R. and Purdie, N. (1998) The attitudes of bilingual children to their languages. *Journal of Multilingual and Multicultural Development* 19 (3), 199–211.

Oller, D.K. (2005) The distributed characteristic in bilingual learning. In J. Cohen, K.T. McAlister, K. Rolstad and J. MacSwan (eds) *Proceedings of the 4th International Symposium on Bilingualism* (pp. 1744–1749). Somerville, MA: Cascadilla Press.

Oller, D.K. and Eilers, R.E. (2002) *Language and Literacy in Bilingual Children*. Clevedon: Multilingual Matters.

Paradis, J. (2004) On the relevance of specific language impairment to understanding the role of transfer in second language acquisition. *Applied Psycholinguistics* 25, 67–82.

Paradis, J. (2005) Grammatical morphology in children learning English as a second language: Implications of similarities with Specific Language Impairment. *Language, Speech and Hearing Services in the Schools* 36, 172–187.

Paradis, J. (2010a) Bilingual children's acquisition of English verb morphology: Effects of language exposure, structure complexity, and task type. *Language Learning* 60 (3), 651–680.

Paradis, J. (2010b) The interface between bilingual development and specific language impairment. Keynote article. *Applied Psycholinguistics* 31, 227–252.

Paradis, J. and Genesee, F. (1996) Syntactic acquisition in bilingual children: Autonomous or interdependent? *Studies in Second Language Acquisition* 18, 1–25.

Paradis, J., Nicoladis, E. and Crago, M. (2007) French-English bilingual children's acquisition of the past tense. In H. Caunt-Nulton, S. Kulatilake and I-H. Woo (eds) *BUCLD 31: Proceedings of the 31st Annual Boston University Conference on Language Development* (pp. 497–507). Somerville, MA: Cascadilla Press.

Paradis, J., Tremblay, A. and Crago, M. (2008) Bilingual children's acquisition of English inflection: The role of language dominance and task type. *BUCLD 32: Proceedings of the 32nd Annual Boston University Conference on Language Development* (Vol. 2; pp. 378–389). Somerville, MA: Cascadilla Press.

Pearson, B.Z., Fernández, S.C., Lewedeg, V. and Oller, D.K. (1997) The relation of input factors to lexical learning by bilingual infants. *Applied Psycholinguistics* 18, 41–58.

Pearson, B.Z., Fernández, S. and Oller, D.K. (1993) Lexical development in bilingual infants and toddlers: Comparison to monolingual norms. *Language Learning* 43, 93–120.

Ramírez, J., Pasta, D., Yuen, S., Ramey, D. and Billings, D. (1991) *Longitudinal Study of Structured English Immersion Strategy. Early-exit and Late-exit Transitional Bilingual Education Programs for Language-minority Children* (Vol. 2). Washington, DC: US Department of Education.

Rhys, M. and Thomas, E.M. (2012) Bilingual Welsh-English children's acquisition of vocabulary and reading: Implications for bilingual education. *International Journal of Bilingual Education and Bilingualism*. DOI: 10.1080/13670050.2012.706248.

Romaine, S. (1995) *Bilingualism*. London: Blackwell.

Thomas, E.M. (2007) The role of the child in language transmission: Child interviews. In V.C.M. Gathercole (ed.) *Language Transmission in Bilingual Families in Wales* (pp. 248–286). Cardiff: Welsh Language Board.

Thomas, E.M., Lewis, W.G. and Apolloni, D. (2012) Variation in language choice in extended speech in primary schools in Wales: Implications for teacher education. *Language and Education* 26 (3), 245–261.

Thomas, E.M. and Roberts, D.B. (2011) Exploring bilinguals' social use of language inside and out of the minority language classroom. *Language and Education* 25 (2), 89–198.

Thomas, E.M., Williams, N.C., Jones, Ll.A., Davies, S. and Binks, H. (under review) Acquiring complex structures under conditions of minimal exposure: Bilingual acquisition of plural morphology in Welsh. *Bilingualism: Language and Cognition*.

Thomas, H. (2010) *Brwydr i Baradwys? Y Dylanwadau as Dwf Ysgolion Cymraeg De-ddwyrain Cymru*. Cardiff: University of Wales Press.

Thordardottir, E. (2011) The relationship between bilingual exposure and vocabulary development. *International Journal of Bilingualism* 15 (4), 426–445.

Thordardottir, E., Rothenberg, A., Rivard, M.E. and Naves, R. (2006) Bilingual assessment: Can overall proficiency be estimated from separate measurement of two languages? *Journal of Multilingual Communication Disorders* 4 (1), 1–21.

Umbel, V.C., Pearson, B.Z., Fernández, M.C. and Oller, D.K. (1992) Measuring bilingual children's receptive vocabularies. *Child Development* 63, 1012–1020.

Vihman, M.M. (1998) A developmental perspective on code-switching: Conversations between a pair of bilingual siblings. *International Journal of Bilingualism* 2, 45–84.

Wei, L. (2000) *The Bilingualism Reader.* London: Routledge.

Welsh Government (2010) Strategaeth Addysg Cyfrwng Cymraeg/Welsh Medium Education Strategy. Cardiff: Welsh Government. http://wales.gov.uk/docs/dcells/publications/100420welshmediumstrategycy.pdf

Welsh Government (2011a) *Welsh Language (Wales) Measure (2011).* Cardiff: Welsh Government.

Welsh Government (2011b) *Welsh Government (2011) Schools Census, 2011: Final Results: General Statistics.* Cardiff: Welsh Government. http://wales.gov.uk/topics/statistics/headlines/schools2011/110906/?skip=1&lang=en

Welsh Language Board (2006) *Young People's Social Networks and Language Use: Final Report.* Cardiff: Welsh Language Board.

10 The Effects of Peer Feedback Practices in Spanish Second Language Writing

Eva Rodríguez-González

The present study examined the impact of peer feedback practices on second language (L2) Spanish writing. Previous research has shown that peer feedback processes enhance audience awareness and facilitate L2 acquisition (Byrd, 1994). However, careful preparation and training are essential for successful peer responses (Stanley, 1992). The investigation involved the participation of 48 students enrolled in three sections of an L2 Spanish composition course: the first section incorporated a two-hour trained peer feedback session; the second did not have a training session but the instructor provided basic guidelines for peer feedback; and the third served as a control group with no peer feedback practices. The results show that participants' grades in the trained section were significantly higher than in other sections. Overall, L2 learners did not feel confident when providing feedback on grammatical accuracy. However, peer comments on content and organization induced more revisions. Despite the amount of work, 94% of the participants were satisfied with the peer feedback and multiple draft approach employed. Additionally, qualitative results suggest that students benefit from reading and revising a draft as it allows them to develop and self-assess their own writing. Implications of these findings for L2 learning theories are also discussed.

The potential benefits of peer feedback in writing at the college level is an area that has occupied the attention of both first language (L1) and second language (L2) teaching, in addition to research on second language acquisition (SLA). Historically, the field of L2 writing has focused primarily on the teaching of writing to English second language writers (Matsuda & De Pew, 2002). More precisely, response activities to student writing in both L1 and L2 college settings have been a persistent topic of discussion (Leki, 1990;

Silva & Brice, 2004). In traditional L2 classrooms, instructors have been the only source that reflects and responds to student writing. However, peer feedback (also referred to as 'peer review', 'peer response', 'peer revision' and 'peer tutoring') is currently viewed as a prominent feature of process-oriented, learner-based instruction (Hyland & Hyland, 2006).

Regarding the effectiveness of such peer feedback methods within L2 contexts, research based on theoretical foundations has provided substantial evidence that the practice of peer feedback significantly contributes to L2 learners' development of their L2 writing abilities. For more than a decade, the practice of peer response has been present in both L1 and L2 writing courses, finding strong support from Vygotsky's sociocultural theory of learning (1962, 1978), Process-Writing Theory in L2 (Kroll, 1991; Mangelsdorf, 1989) and Bruffee's Collaborative Learning Theory (1993). In sociocultural approaches, language development is viewed as a social process that requires social interaction. Under this conception, knowledge is not sustained solely by the L2 learner as an individual, but also by the contextual and social settings in which it is used. The importance of that contextual environment is shown in research that examines learners' success in L2 classroom peer interaction where learners are able to help one another as they interact (Donato, 1994; Ohta, 2001). Thus, development is visible through microgenetic analyses of episodes of interaction (Lantolf, 2000; Ohta, 2001). In relation to sociocultural theories, Ohta (2001) found that adult learners of Japanese in their first two years of language instruction helped each other with a variety of tasks that incorporated peer interaction. Similarly, Swain (2001) found that French immersion students working in pairs in writing activities reflected consciously on the language they were producing as they provided assistance to their peers. In both studies, learner collaboration was primarily related to language form. By means of receiving and providing assistance, a learner discourse of joint performance emerges as a way of anticipating individual production (Foster & Ohta, 2005).

Continuing with a sociocultural perspective, the zone of proximal development (ZPD) has been identified to account for the relationship between assistance and language development. Vygotsky (1978) defined the ZPD as the distance between the actual developmental level and the level of potential development. While Vygotsky originally developed the notion of the ZPD to account for children's development, his theoretical framework has been employed by L2 researchers such as Donato (1994) and Lantolf and Appel (1994) to investigate interaction in group activities examining how peer feedback in the L2 writing classroom influences language learning. Ohta (2001) articulated the ZPD for L2 learning as 'the distance between the actual developmental level as determined by individual linguistic production, and the level of potential development as determined through language produced collaboratively with a teacher or a peer' (Ohta, 2001: 9). The specific implications of the ZPD for SLA suggest that language development occurs as the gap between individual and collaborative performance is filled and learners develop increased independence.

More specific to L2 writing, process-writing theory in L2 focuses on the process of writing, viewing writing not as a product-based activity but rather as one that is both dynamic and recursive (Kroll, 1991; Mangelsdorf, 1989). In L2 classroom settings, peer feedback supports process writing with a focus on drafting and revision that enables students to receive multiple types of feedback (from instructor and peers) across various drafts. Furthermore, peer feedback builds audience awareness and allows connections to be made between reading and writing through multiple exposures to a given text. Finally, research in L1 writing has also found a plethora of benefits of employing collaborative learning techniques in the classroom. Research studies have found that in writing groups students negotiate meaning as they help each other revise their writings (Gere, 1987) and that learning in writing groups is a reciprocal process that improves students' work (Bruffee, 1984; Hirvela, 1999). As Bruffee (1984) maintains, while students individually may not have all the knowledge or resources available to successfully complete a task, 'pooling the resources that a group of peers brings with them to the task' (Bruffee, 1984: 644) may enable the group to complete a task that individuals may not be able to complete on their own.

Aligned with the potential advantages that peer feedback has been shown to offer in L2 writing, a significant amount of research literature has also identified a number of challenges associated with the implementation of peer feedback in an L2 course. First, L2 students' limited knowledge of the target language is considered the main source of difficulty for helping one another (Villamil & de Guerrero, 1996). Similarly, L2 student writers may also lack the ability to distinguish valuable and non-valuable feedback (Leki, 1990; Stanley, 1992) and to revise their own writing according to the comments provided by peers (Connor & Asenavage, 1994; Liu & Sadler, 2003). There is also the issue of the nature of peer feedback strategies employed. L2 students seem to focus on surface language concerns in their peer reviews (Leki, 1990), and they tend to provide vague comments (Liu & Sadler, 2003) or what Stanley (1992: 219) refers to as 'rubber stamp advice', such as 'be more specific'. Finally, it is important to acknowledge that peer readers are sometimes reluctant to provide comments on other students' writing. Students may fear ridiculing their peers for their foreign language problems (Nelson & Carson, 1998). Added to the fact that students may question their ability as efficient peer feedback providers, there is a strong tendency in students to trust the instructor more than their peers. In this regard, it has been documented that university students prefer instructor feedback to feedback from peers and are much more likely to incorporate it in their future revisions (Nelson & Carson, 1998).

For peer feedback to become a successful and efficient strategy that will contribute to the improvement of L2 writing skills, explicit instructor intervention may be necessary. This intervention can help to increase student motivation and understanding of the potential advantages of peer feedback as an additional source of feedback aside from instructor feedback. In this regard, one perspective that examines ways of improving the quality of written peer feedback is the incorporation of training and preparation in the L2 curriculum. The role of training in L2 writing has been investigated through the hypothesis that explicit instructor-based guidance through the mechanism of collaborative learning can influence the quality of L2 student writing. According to Stanley (1992), careful preparation and training are essential for successful peer response. Stanley found that a group of university English foreign language (EFL) students trained in peer evaluation offered more feedback and couched it more tactfully than an untrained control group. Student writers were also more likely to use the feedback provided by trained peers in their revisions. Min (2005) conducted a classroom-based study to train students on how to provide peer feedback in an L2 English writing setting. Her results revealed that L2 learners produced significantly more comments and were able to produce more relevant and specific comments on global issues in the text after being coached to be successful reviewers than an uncoached control group did. In a subsequent study, Min (2006) examined the impact of trained responders' feedback on EFL college students' revisions. After a four-hour in-class demonstration and a one-hour after-class reviewer–instructor conference with each student, results showed that students incorporated a significantly higher number of reviewers' comments into their revisions after the peer review training. The results obtained by Zhu (1995) also reported that peer feedback training had a significant effect on both the quantity and quality of feedback. Other researchers have also found that students who have been trained in peer response tend to provide more useful feedback to their peers (Berg, 1999; Hyland & Hyland, 2006; Paulus, 1999). Additionally, training and careful preparation can benefit student reviewers themselves as they are in a better position to view their own texts from a reader's perspective (Ferris, 2003; Hyland, 2003). In summary, peer feedback training interventions in L2 curricula are conceptualized as a trigger for L2 learners to expand their understanding of the target language by seeing and evaluating both successful and unsuccessful language production strategies through their peers.

The Present Study

The present study continues the work that existing research studies have accomplished by examining the impact and effectiveness of explicit L2 peer feedback training techniques in L2 course design. By incorporating previous work, the present study builds upon the findings that identify the

198 Solutions for the Assessment of Bilinguals

advantages of using trained peer feedback procedures to enhance L2 output skills such as writing. This study focuses on intermediate L2 Spanish learners, a group beyond the novice language level that is characterized as having strong features of *interlanguage* (Selinker, 1972) development. This study incorporates peer feedback into a process of writing multiple draft revisions in an intermediate Spanish conversation course at a college level. Two different experimental groups involving peer feedback activities are compared with a control group that did not engage in peer feedback practices. Additionally, the Spanish course selected for the study uses a retrospective evaluation protocol to determine to what extent peer feedback activities enhance language awareness and build self-confidence and perceived language competence in L2 writing. The study attempts to determine to what extent students benefit from the practice of substantial trained peer feedback to improve L2 Spanish writing skills. To that end, the following research questions are addressed:

(1) *Efficacy.* Does peer feedback positively impact L2 Spanish learners' writing? Does the implementation of explicit training interventions facilitate peer feedback?
(2) *Learner acceptance.* What perceptions do L2 learners generally hold toward peer feedback after its practice? What are the salient factors that determine the L2 learners' perceptions of peer feedback?
(3) *Student versus instructor impacts.* What are the respective roles played by instructor and peer comments in peer feedback practices in L2 Spanish writing?

Method

Participants

Forty-eight Spanish L2 learners (28% male and 72% female) were recruited from three different sections of a third-year Intermediate Spanish Grammar Review and Composition course at a Midwestern university in the United States. Participants had to be present for each phase of the experiment in order to be included in the investigation. Two sections of the course, Sections A and B ($n = 14$ and 16, respectively), were assigned as experimental groups and the third section, Section C ($n = 18$), as the control group. All three sections of the course were taught by the same instructor to eliminate potential differences in teaching styles (the instructor of the course was not the researcher of the present study). All participants were native speakers of English and had been exposed to formal Spanish instruction in classroom settings before enrolling on the course. All of them had either taken a Spanish course previously to the one reported in this study at the same institution or had been placed in the course through a Spanish language placement exam. Based on placement test scores, previous experience with Spanish and informal observations, participants in the study can be broadly categorized as intermediate language learners as described by the proficiency guidelines of the American Council of Teaching Foreign Languages (ACTFL, 2012). These students exhibit the hallmarks of intermediate level proficiency according to the following criteria of the ACTFL Proficiency Guidelines: They can communicate simple facts and ideas in a loosely connected series of sentences on topics of personal interest and social needs in the present. They can express meaning through vocabulary and basic structures that are comprehensible to those accustomed to the writing of non-native speakers (Breiner-Sanders *et al.*, 2001).

The course was a requirement for Spanish majors and it was the first in a sequence of courses that focused primarily on writing skills. The course met three times per week throughout a five-month semester. None of the participants had been exposed to peer feedback in foreign language courses prior to the study. However, all the participants enrolled on the course had been exposed in previous courses to the one-draft one-reader (instructor) writing practice that placed much emphasis on grammatical accuracy.

Design and procedure

As a regular practice in the L2 course, students were expected to submit several writing assignments throughout the semester. For each assignment, students had to submit two drafts. The instructor provided written comments on the first draft; these suggested changes were to be incorporated in the second draft. Thus, the instructor's feedback was present at all stages of the writing process. Students on the course were asked to keep a student writing portfolio to track writing development. Students on the course had to submit all drafts for each assignment in order to track the development of their writing (Hamp-Lyons, 2009). The three sections of the course used the same topic in each of the writing assignments, and each writing assignment was distributed during a 50-minute class session. The course syllabus included monthly writing workshops to help students to focus on writing skills. Each draft of the assignment was weighted equally (50 points per draft, out of 100 total points per assignment) to encourage students to pay attention to the revision process. All writing drafts used in the present study were evaluated using a common rubric by both the instructor of the course and by an independent rater (inter-rater reliability was at 85%, Pearson coefficient correlation value $r = 0.85099$, $p < 0.0001$). The rater used for the present study had previously taught the same course at the institution and was familiar with the teaching practices and materials used in the course. The rubric measured performance in four categories: content (10%), organization (30%), vocabulary (10%), grammar (30%) and spelling/accents (20%). The course instructor provided written comments on the first draft by means of using an error correction code system, in which the instructor highlighted a word/sentence using a specific symbol so that the student knew that an error

needed to be corrected (cf. Appendix A), but students were tasked with identifying how to alter the highlighted text on their own. For instance, the
instructor underlined a sentence to indicate problems with paragraph organization or circled a word to indicate a spelling error. Students were provided
with both the evaluation rubric and the error correction codes before the
writing assignments were due.

The research study was conducted over the span of two months and incorporated the entire process of two writing assignments as well as the completion of pre- and post-implementation questionnaires. At the very beginning
of the research study, a short language history survey was distributed to assess
previous experience in Spanish as well as other factors such as age and gender.
Participants were also asked some questions about previous exposure to
Spanish writing practices. Questions on the background questionnaire are
based on those in a study by Tsui and Ng (2000) and focused on students'
attitudes and experience toward writing in previous and current semesters of
study. Participants were asked about their previous exposure to multiple draft
writing approaches and peer feedback practices before enrolling in the course
where the research study took place. With regard to prior experience with
multiple draft processes in writing, 58% of participants had previous experience in general courses. However, only 17% of participants reported having
been exposed to multiple draft writing processes in a foreign language course.
In terms of prior exposure to peer feedback practices, 7% of participants had
been engaged in peer feedback in general courses, but none of them had been
provided with guidelines to check their peers' writing samples. Additionally,
none of the participants in the present study reported experience in providing
and receiving peer feedback in writing assignments in a foreign language
course. These patterns of results do not differ across the three groups of the
Spanish course that have been chosen for the present study. That is, the three
groups were equated in terms of previous exposure with multiple draft and
peer feedback practices before the present study was introduced.

After completing the language survey and background questionnaire,
participants submitted their first assignment with two drafts. The instructor provided feedback on the first assignment. The student re-wrote the
essay and returned a polished draft for a grade. The second submission constituted the final version of the assignment. Each writing cycle in the research
course lasted four weeks and began with a brainstorming activity involving
the entire class before the production of each piece of writing. The production of a first draft followed and a week later the instructor gave whole-class
feedback on common problems as well as providing individual written comments and grades to each student. Based on the written and oral comments
provided by the instructor, students revised their drafts to produce a final
second version of the assignment. The second writing cycle was different in
Sections A and B of the present study because peer feedback was provided
together with instructor feedback. Thus, right after the submission of a first

draft, both instructor and peers provided written and oral comments (there was a peer response session of 15 minutes where two peers commented among themselves on each other's drafts).

The results from the first assignment (first draft and revised version) were analyzed as a baseline comparison with which to compare the performance on the second assignment (cf. Figure 10.1 in the results section below). The main objective of the first assignment was to familiarize participants with the drafting process, rubrics and instructor's feedback and grading. Once all participants had submitted their second and final draft of their second assignment of the semester, participants in the feedback groups completed a questionnaire about students' perceptions of the usefulness of reading peers' Spanish writings and peers' written comments. Questions in the post-implementation questionnaire were modeled on Tsui and Ng (2000). These questions asked participants about their perceptions of the usefulness of reading peers' writings (items 1–5), the usefulness of reading peers' written comments (items 6–10), the usefulness of the instructor's comments (items 11–15), which aspects of their writing improved after the revisions (items 16–20), and how satisfied participants were with the peer feedback practice used (see Table 10.1 below with each item). In addition, the present study incorporated the questions used in the semi-structured interviews in Tsui and Ng (2000) in a written format. Thus, open-ended questions were added to the first set of 21 Likert-scale items.

Experimental and control sections of the course

Participants in the first experimental group, Section A, attended a trained peer review session of two hours' duration. The training took place outside class time at a day and time agreed upon by the participants and the researcher (author of the present study). The training was conducted right after participants had submitted the first draft of the second writing assignment and before the instructor had provided written comments on the draft. The training activities used in the present study were adopted from Hu (2005) and consisted of the following activities:

(a) *Raising awareness activity.* In groups of three, participants discussed potential advantages and disadvantages of using peer feedback practices in second language courses in order to develop a positive attitude towards the specific teaching strategy employed (Berg, 1999). The entire class engaged in the discussion. The researcher also informed the participants about research findings on the implementation of peer feedback in L2 language courses.

(b) *Demonstration and practice activity.* The researcher selected four anonymous, typed writing samples collected during a previous semester for the same course of the study and showed these to students during the first part of the training session. The sample writings showcased other

Spanish second language learners at similar writing proficiency levels. The first three samples showcased grammar problems that impeded communication (sample 1), ineffective organization due to lack of use of discourse markers (sample 2), and a limited range of vocabulary that limited details in terms of content (sample 3). The fourth sample illustrated grammar problems that did not impede communication, but nevertheless showed effective use of discourse markers to facilitate organization, and diverse vocabulary use that contributed to the detail of information presented in the essay. The ultimate goal of the training was to provide learners with techniques for successful writing. By means of analyzing and critiquing samples, it was hoped that participants in the training session would be able to identify areas of strength and weakness in their own writing and the writing of their peers.

After viewing the initial four samples, the researcher then asked participants to compare the first three training writing samples with the fourth. The session continued on to the analysis of a new fifth writing sample. Participants were divided into pairs to discuss the sample and to identify strengths and weaknesses and write down their comments. Then all participants in the training discussed the fifth writing sample with the researcher in terms of content, organization, vocabulary and grammar. Attention to detail in all of these areas was emphasized in order to help participants provide better feedback on their peers' writing. To conclude this activity, the entire class reflected on appropriate types of responses and effective use of language when providing peer feedback.

(c) *Individual peer feedback activity.* At the end of the training session, the researcher assigned participants a peer feedback activity for which participants had to provide written comments on one of their peers' assignments during the current semester (first draft of the second assignment of the research study). After participants provided written comments to their peers, they met with each other in pairs to talk about their writing and their peers' responses.

Participants in the second experimental group, Section B, were also engaged in peer feedback practices similar to those of the participants in Section A. The difference between the two groups was that participants in Section B were provided only with some basic guidelines as to how to provide peer feedback, but they did not receive any formal training about how to conduct peer feedback.

In contrast with the experimental groups, participants in the control group did not engage in peer feedback practices throughout the semester. Participants in the control group were assigned the same writing prompts and rubrics for assessment purposes but only had instructor comments on their assignments.

Results

Three aspects of the data will be examined: participants' potential improvement on the revisions of each assignment based on difference scores between the second and first drafts; participants' responses on the post-questionnaire; and qualitative feedback from participants in the two sections that involved peer feedback practices.

Grades

The first research question aimed to examine whether peer feedback activities enhanced L2 writing in adult L2 Spanish learners. In order to answer the question, the two experimental groups that incorporated different modalities of peer feedback were compared to the control group. The score submitted for analysis was the difference between the scores in the two versions of the second assignment. Each draft in the assignment constituted 50% of the grade, so the first and second drafts were equally weighted towards the final grade per assignment. Thus, a total of 50 points was possible with a grading scale divided as follows: 30–34 points = D; 35–39 = C; 40–44 = B; 45–50 = A). The graders of the assignments were the instructor and a graduate student who had taught the same course in previous semesters. The researcher (author of the present study) was not involved in the grading activity. The graders did not know which section they were grading or which writing draft corresponded to each participant since all the assignments were assigned a code with no names or other identifiers.

A repeated-measures ANOVA was carried out to examine the interaction between the three treatment groups and writing assignments on difference scores between the first and second drafts of each assignment (see means and standard deviations presented in Figure 10.1 below). The three treatment groups were a between-subjects measure and the two writing assignments were a within-subjects variable. A main effect of treatment group was found, indicating that participants' difference scores were significantly different across the three groups [F (2, 45) = 6.659, p = 0.003]. There was an overall strong tendency towards significance between the two assignments, indicating that participants' performance on the second assignment yielded better results after the peer feedback activities were introduced in the course, [F (1, 45) = 3.066, p = 0.087]. There was also a statistically significant interaction between assignments and treatment groups [F (2, 45) = 4.212, p = 0.021]. In the first assignment, before the peer feedback intervention took place, no significant differences were found across the three treatment groups [F (2, 45) = 0.666, p = 0.519]. However, there were statistically significant differences across the three treatment groups in the second assignment after the peer feedback intervention.

Participants' difference scores in the section that incorporated trained peer feedback were significantly higher than those in the control group,

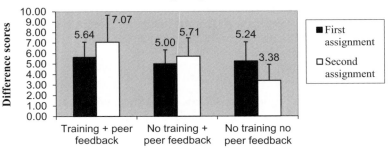

Figure 10.1 Means and standard deviations in participants' difference scores in the first and second writing assignments across the three treatment groups. Difference scores were obtained by calculating grades for the second draft minus those for the first draft per each writing assignment. Means for each condition are shown above each bar

$p = 0.001$, difference scores for participants in the non-coached peer feedback section were also significantly different from those in the control group, $p = 0.003$, and there was a strong tendency for difference scores in the trained peer feedback group to be higher than those in the non-trained peer feedback group, $p = 0.06$. Thus, the results indicate that the implementation of peer feedback practices positively enhanced the quality of L2 Spanish writing from an initial to a polished draft.

Questionnaire data

Apart from objective measurements of increased language performance in L2 Spanish writing as attested in assignment grades, the study also included an analysis of L2 learners' perceptions about the usefulness of peer feedback practices. Only participants in the peer feedback groups (groups A and B) filled out a questionnaire, since the control group was not exposed to peer feedback activities. Responses were grouped according to four constructs, namely: (i) participants' perception of the usefulness of reading peers' writings (Items 1–5); (ii) the usefulness of peers' comments (Items 6–10); (iii) the usefulness of the instructor's comments (Items 11–15); and (iv) the usefulness of the overall peer revision process (Items 16–20). Participants were asked to respond on a Likert scale of 1 to 5, with 1 indicating strong disagreement and 5 indicating strong agreement with the statements (see Table 10.1 for the mean scores and standard deviations of all the items included in the questionnaire).

The overall means for the usefulness were: (i) reading peers' writing, 3.77; (ii) receiving peers' comments, 3.33; (iii) instructor's comments, 4.69; and (iv) peer revision process, 4.38. With the exception of Item 9 in Table 10.1 ($p = 0.861$), the mean values for all the items on the questionnaire were statistically larger than the neutral value of 3, indicating that, on average,

Table 10.1 Post-implementation questionnaire about participants' perceptions of the usefulness of peer feedback practices: Descriptive statistics and mean comparisons for self-assessment values for groups A and B

		M (S.D.)
1.	I find reading my peers' writing samples useful	3.53 (1.11)
2.	Reading my peers' writing samples gave me more ideas	3.90 (0.76)
3.	Reading my peers' compositions helped me to improve the organization of my own composition	3.63 (0.81)
4.	Reading my peers' compositions helped me to improve the language (grammar and vocabulary) of my composition	3.66 (0.88)
5.	I benefited from reading my peers' compositions	3.93 (0.69)
6.	I found my classmates' comments useful	3.60 (0.81)
7.	My classmates' comments helped me to enrich the content of my composition	3.53 (1.00)
8.	My classmates' comments helped me to improve the organization of my composition	3.37 (0.85)
9.	My classmates' comments helped me to improve the language (including grammar and vocabulary) of my composition	3.03 (1.03)
10.	I benefited from my classmates' comments	3.33 (0.88)
11.	I found my instructor's comments useful	4.33 (0.80)
12.	My instructor's comments helped me to enrich the content of my composition	4.33 (1.09)
13.	My instructor's comments helped me to improve the organization of my composition	3.86 (0.82)
14.	My instructor's comments helped me to improve the language (including grammar and vocabulary) of my composition	4.67 (0.61)
15.	I benefited from my instructor's comments	4.60 (0.49)
16.	My composition became better after revisions	4.70 (0.53)
17.	After each revision, the content of my composition became richer	4.27 (0.78)
18.	After each revision, the organization of my writing sample became richer	3.93 (0.78)
19.	After each revision, the Spanish language (grammar and vocabulary) of my writing sample improved	4.47 (0.51)
20.	Revisions helped improve my composition	4.67 (0.48)
21.	I hope that my Spanish instructor/s will continue to use this approach to teach writing in other courses	4.47 (0.68)

Note: Participants responded to all these items on a five-point Likert scale ranging from 1 (strongly disagree) to 5 (strongly agree), with the midpoint value of 3 labeled as neutral.

participants agreed with all of the statements (cf. Figure 10.2 below). A repeated-measures ANOVA was conducted, with treatment groups A and B as between-subjects measure and the different sets of items as within-subjects variables. There was no main effect of treatment group, indicating that participants' perceptions about the use of peer feedback practices were similar in the two groups [F (1, 28) = 0.117, p = 0.735]. But there was a significant main effect of question type, [F (1, 28) = 61.020, $p < 0.001$]. Participants found that instructor's comments were the most helpful aspect of the feedback process [F (1, 28) = 9.290, p = 0.005].

Results from the post-implementation questionnaire show that participants felt that reading peers' L2 Spanish writings helped them identify their own strengths and put them into perspective when improving their own writing (Items 1–5). They also perceived that peer comments helped them to enrich the content and organization of their L2 writing (Items 6–10). However, they did not believe that their L2 writing improved in the areas of grammar and vocabulary from peers' comments (Item 9). However, participants noticed that their L2 writing samples improved after revision (Item 16), with the assistance of both peer (Item 6) and instructor feedback (Item 11). Furthermore, participants remarked that content, organization and grammar functions were positively influenced by the dynamics of the revision process employed in the course writing assignment (Items 17–20). The writing sample revision process suggests that this procedure may be one way to effectively improve participants' self-perceptions of their own writing in L2 Spanish.

When examining the relative value of reviewer feedback, the results obtained for Items 9 and 14 indicate that participants prefer the instructor's feedback for attaining grammatical accuracy. Instructors are valued as authoritative figures in the learning process in classroom settings in terms of knowledge of the subject matter, experience, and advanced proficiency in the L2

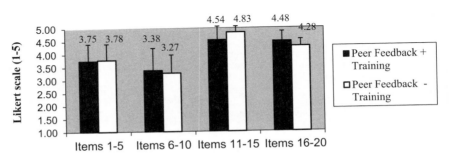

Figure 10.2 Means and standard deviations in participants' perceptions of the usefulness of peer feedback practices in L2 Spanish writing. Means for each condition are shown above each bar

language. Finally, the results also suggest a high degree of participant satisfaction (94%) regarding the process-drafting and peer feedback procedures that were used in the course (Item 21). Results from Items 6, 10, 16 and 20 indicate that participants attributed learning value to the strategies used in the course.

Qualitative responses

Qualitative data in the form of open-ended questions in the questionnaire also reveal positive findings. When asked about preference for specific types of peer comments, 97% of the participants identified content and organization as the main factors that they found most valuable from peers. In this regard, one of the participants indicated that s/he 'preferred comments about content since the teacher focuses on grammar and vocabulary'. Similarly, there were seven instances where participants signaled specific types of peer feedback: 'those comments [peers'] and opinions really helped on the content part, where the teacher did not comment as much'. In terms of identifying potential benefits from receiving and giving comments to peers, it was common to find comments made by participants in both experimental groups (trained peer feedback and non-coached peer feedback sections) that referred to self-evaluation mechanisms such as the following: '[receiving comments from peers] made me examine my own composition with a fresh and realistic perspective . . . Giving comments to others allowed me to see the level at which they write at as well as helped me realize that I am capable of editing for content or organization in Spanish.' Some of the participants, however, identified a lack of confidence when providing peer feedback in L2 writing because of L2 language proficiency: 'I did not really benefit from giving them [peer comments], because I feel I am not the best judge for Spanish for others.' Finally, all participants in the experimental groups identified a clear preference for the instructor's comments in terms of grammar because the instructor's comments are 'always right. They [instructors] are the graders. I want their opinions the most.'

In summary, participants in groups A and B positively valued peer feedback activities and self-perceived an increase in written L2 Spanish language performance after the peer feedback process was implemented. Peer comments were considered to be valuable resources, but specific roles were assigned when evaluating the preference and usefulness of comments provided. The degree of satisfaction with the practice of peer feedback activities was sufficiently high that participants expressed the desire to continue with peer feedback practices and other writing activities in the future (cf. Item 21 in Table 10.1).

Discussion

This study examined the impact that peer feedback activities can have on L2 Spanish writing. The results of the experiment demonstrated that L2 learners can indeed benefit from collaborative learning despite the fact that they perceive a certain degree of inability to provide comments on their peers' L2 language production. More specifically, the results in the present study tend to favor a coached teaching intervention on how to provide successful peer feedback despite L2 self-perceived lack of competence. Participants found it useful to read and provide comments on their peers' writing as a way not only to provide feedback to their peers but also to improve their own individual writing. They identified a learning value in peers' comments as part of raising awareness of the strengths and weaknesses of their own L2 writing. The fact that participants in the peer feedback group that did not receive training (group B) also identified positive awareness raising effects suggests that awareness raising of different kinds of writing issues is not solely connected with the training session that participants in group A received. However, it could be reasonable to consider that the training itself made learners more aware of specific aspects of their own writing and that may have resulted in an improvement of their writing separately from the peer feedback practice itself. Although instructor feedback was preferred for grammatical accuracy, L2 learners identified a positive impact of their peers' feedback in their L2 writing in terms of content and organization. This study suggests a role for instructors to incorporate peer feedback practices as a way to facilitate L2 learners' progress in their writing process.

These findings are in line with theoretical approaches that identify the value of peer feedback procedures. In the present study, peer feedback practices had a prominent place in process-oriented writing instruction since these practices involved participants' reading, critiquing and writing, both to secure immediate textual improvement and to enhance writing competence through mutual scaffolding (Hu, 2005; Tsui & Ng, 2000; Zhu, 2001). In addition to process-based learning, the present study also supports the theoretical views that are formulated in Vygotsky's sociocultural theory of learning (1962, 1978) and sociocognitive approaches. Both self-confidence and self-efficacy as socially and cognitively defined constructs are influenced by collaborative procedures among L2 learners as key factors in one's ability to learn an L2 and seek intercultural communication. By means of engaging in peer feedback activities, L2 learners' perceived competence increases as they perceive themselves as being able to successfully provide and comment upon other L2 learners' writing (Baker & MacIntyre, 2003). L2 learners' retrospective evaluations on the potential learning value of peer feedback practices become crucial to exercising control over thoughts and future actions. The findings reported on the post-implementation questionnaire in the present study suggest that participants felt that they benefited from both reading and providing comments to their peers' L2 writing in Spanish.

Although the present study shows the significant contributions of peer feedback activities to L2 language learning, the claims made on the basis of these data regarding the effects of peer feedback for long-term implications are tentative. One issue that will need to be addressed in future research is that of time. The current study was conducted over a relatively short period of time. It would be of interest to determine how long any effects from the peer feedback process persist over a longer time frame. Future research should also continue to investigate the details of negotiations that occur during L2 peer feedback practices and the ways these negotiations shape L2 learners' revision activities and self-awareness. Finally, a future study should separate the group that provided feedback with a specific training intervention on how to provide peer feedback from a group who received feedback per se, in order to determine which is more important in influencing the L2 learners' performance in writing.

To conclude, the present study informs ecologically valid classroom research, so that instructors may eventually have a pedagogical tool that can be used to enhance the classroom environment. This study also emphasizes the importance of empowering L2 learners in their capabilities of learning and helping their peers through exposure to different kinds of L2 writing and meta-analysis procedures. Should instructors incorporate peer feedback activities in their L2 courses, L2 learners will be more actively engaged in their L2 language learning and will more likely seek out different ways of learning under a contextualized learning environment. Ultimately, peer feedback procedures will encourage a more reflective and active response in L2 learners that will allow for raising awareness not only of writing conventions themselves, but also of developing and improving learning and overall language acquisition.

Acknowledgements

This research was supported by an Assessment Grant from the Office of Liberal Education and Assessment at Miami University of Ohio, USA. Special thanks are due to Catherine Bishop-Clark and Beth Uhler for their thoughtful comments and suggestions. The author also thanks the instructor of the course at the time the study was conducted, Martin Kane, and the outside-instructor rater, Anneris Coria-Navia, for their time and support of the project.

References

ACTFL (American Council on the Teaching of Foreign Languages) (2012) *ACTFL Proficiency Guidelines*. Alexandria, VA: ACTFL.

Baker, S.C. and MacIntyre, P.D. (2003) The role of gender and immersion in immersion and second language orientations. *Language Learning* 53, 65–96.

Berg, E.C. (1999) The effects of trained peer response on ESL students' revision types and writing quality. *Journal of Second Language Writing* 8, 215–241.

Breiner-Sanders, K.E., Swender, E. and Terry, R.M. (2001) *Preliminary Proficiency Guidelines – Writing: Revised*. Hastings-on-Hudson, NY: ACTFL Materials Center.

Bruffee, K. (1984) Collaborative learning and the conversation of mankind. *College English* 46, 635–652.

Bruffee, K. (1993) *Collaborative Learning: Higher Education, Interdependence, and the Authority of Knowledge*. Baltimore, MD: Johns Hopkins University Press.

Byrd, D.R. (1994) Peer editing: Common concerns and applications in the foreign language classroom. *Die Unterrichtsprzxis/Teaching German* 21, 119–123.

Connor, U. and Asenavage, K. (1994) Peer response groups in ESL writing classes: How much impact on revision? *Journal of Second Language Writing* 3, 257–275.

Donato, R. (1994) Collective scaffolding in second language acquisition. In J.P. Lantolf and G. Appel (eds) *Vygotskian Approaches to Second Language Research*. Norwood, NJ: Ablex.

Ferris, D.R. (2003) Responding to writing. In B. Kroll (ed.) *Exploring the Dynamics of Second Language Writing* (pp. 119–140). Cambridge: Cambridge University Press.

Foster, P. and Ohta, A.S. (2005) Negotiation for meaning and peer assistance in second language classrooms. *Applied Linguistics* 26, 402–430.

Gere, A. (1987) Writing groups: History, theory, and communication. *Studies in Writing and Rhetoric*. Carbondale, IL: Illinois University Press.

Hamp-Lyons, L. (2009) The challenges of second-language writing assessment. In B. Huot and P. O'Neill (eds) *Assessing Writing: A Critical Sourcebook*. NCTE with Bedford/ St. Martins. Originally published in E.M. White, W.D. Lutz and S. Kamusikiri (eds) (1996) *Assessment of Writing: Politics, Policies, Practices* (pp. 226–240). NY: MLA. Reprinted by permission of the Modern Language Association.

Hirvela, A. (1999) Collaborative writing: Instruction and communities of readers and writers. *TESOL Journal* 8, 7–12.

Hu, G. (2005) Using peer review with Chinese ESL student writers. *Language Teaching Research* 9, 312–342.

Hyland, F. (2003) Focusing on form: Student engagement with teacher feedback. *System* 31, 217–230.

Hyland, K. and Hyland, F. (2006) *Feedback on Second Language Students' Writing. Contexts and Issues*. Cambridge: Cambridge University Press.

Kroll, B. (1991) Teaching writing in the ESL context. In M. Celce-Murcia (ed.) *Teaching English as a Second or Foreign Language* (2nd edn; pp. 245–263). New York: Newbury House/Harper Collins.

Lantolf, J.P. (2000) *Sociocultural Theory and Second Language Learning*. Oxford: Oxford University Press.

Lantolf, J.P. and Appel, G. (1994) *Vygotskian Approaches to Second Language Research*. Norwood, NJ: Ablex.

Leki, I. (1990) Coaching from the margins: Issues in written response. In B. Kroll (ed.) *Second Language Writing* (pp. 57–68). Cambridge: Cambridge University Press.

Liu, J. and Sadler, R.W. (2003) The effect and affect of peer review in electronic versus traditional modes on L2 writing. *Journal of English for Academic Purposes* 2, 193–227.

Mangelsdorf, K. (1989) Parallels between speaking and writing in second language acquisition. In D. Johnson and D. Roen (eds) *Richness in Writing: Empowering ESL Students* (pp. 134–135). White Plains, NY: Longman.

Matsuda, P.K. and De Pew, K.E. (2002) Early second language writing: An introduction. *Journal of Second Language Writing* 11, 261–268.

Min, H.T. (2005) Training students to become successful peer reviewers. *System* 33, 293–308.

Min, H.T. (2006) The effects of trained peer review on EFL students' revision types and writing quality. *Journal of Second Language Writing* 5, 118–141.

Nelson, G. and Carson, J.G. (1998) ESL students' perceptions of effectiveness in peer response groups. *Journal of Second Language Writing 7*, 113–131.

Ohta, A.S. (2001) *Second Language Acquisition Processes in the Classroom: Learning Japanese.* Mahwah, NJ: Lawrence Erlbaum.

Paulus, T.M. (1999) The effect of peer and teacher feedback on student writing. *Journal of Second Language Writing 3*, 265–289.

Selinker, L. (1972) Interlanguage. *International Review of Applied Linguistics* 10, 209–230.

Silva, T. and Brice, C. (2004) Research in teaching writing. *Annual Review of Applied Linguistics* 24, 70–106.

Stanley, J. (1992) Coaching student writers to be effective peer evaluators. *Journal of Second Language Writing* 1 (3), 217–233.

Swain, M. (2001) Integrating language and content teaching through collaborative tasks. *Canadian Modern Language Review* 58, 44–63.

Tsui, A.B.M. and Ng, M. (2000) Do secondary L2 writers benefit from peer comments? *Journal of Second Language Writing 9*, 147–170.

Villamil, O.S. and De Guerrero, M. (1996) Peer revision in the L2 classroom: Social-cognitive activities, mediating strategies, and aspects of social behavior. *Journal of Second Language Writing 3*, 51–75.

Vygotsky, L.S. (1962) *Thought and Language*. Cambridge, MA: MIT Press.

Vygotsky, L.S. (1978) Interaction between language learning and development. In M. Cole, V. John-Steiner, S. Scribner and E. Souberman (eds) *Mind in Society: The Development of Higher Psychological Processes* (pp. 79–91). Cambridge, MA: Harvard University Press.

Zhu, W. (1995) Effects of training for peer response on students' comments and interaction. *Written Communication* 12, 492–528.

Zhu, W. (2001) Interaction and feedback in mixed peer response groups. *Journal of Second Language Writing* 10, 251–276.

Appendix A: Error Correction Code Used in the Present Study for Writing Assignments

Area	Symbol used by instructor	Description
Content	_____?	Content not clear (reader has problems understanding the content)
Vocabulary	(oval)	False cognate
		Dictionary error
		Word choice
		Wrong verb
Grammar/ language use	(rectangle)	Missing a word
		Extra word (not needed)
		Incorrect gender assignment to a noun

Area	Symbol used by instructor	Description
		Incorrect number assignment to a noun
		Concordance (agreement gender/ number with nouns and adjectives)
		Por/para confusion
		Direct/indirect object pronouns
		Personal 'a'
		Contraction error: al, del, conmigo, contigo …
		Prepositional error
		Omission of definite article
		Subject-verb agreement
		Conjugation of a verb
		Preterite imperfect confusion
		Verb tense error (other than preterite-imperfect)
		Reflexive
		Participle error
		'Gustar and similar constructions' error
		Ser/estar/haber confusion
		Incorrect mode (confusion among indicative-subjunctive-infinitive)
		Subjunctive: present should be past or vice versa
		Impersonal 'se' – passive voice
		Missing a verb
		Syntax (wrong word order)
		Not a sentence in Spanish
Spelling	～～～～～～～～	Accent
		Spelling error

11 Commentary on *Issues in the Assessment of Bilinguals* and *Solutions for the Assessment of Bilinguals*

Erika Hoff

Accurate assessment of children's language knowledge is crucially important, and it is also extraordinarily difficult. Assessment has important consequences in multiple domains: assessments of children's language skills are used in basic research, in educational placement, in program evaluation and in clinical diagnosis (Barrueco *et al.*, 2012). Assessment is difficult because language knowledge must be inferred from indirect and imperfect indicators in observable behavior. For children who are bilingual, the difficulty of assessment is greater still. The chapters in these timely books take up the topic of how to assess language and literacy in bilinguals as the need to do so is burgeoning.

There is a growing demand for instruments and procedures to assess bilingual children from researchers, educators and clinicians. The increased demand from research reflects the recognition in scientific circles that bilingualism is not a rare variation on the normative case of monolingual development. Rather, dual language exposure is a normal experience and bilingual development a normal outcome, which any theory of language acquisition needs to be able to handle. In addition, findings from the study of bilingual children have shown that bilingual development provides a unique window onto the nature of human language acquisition capacity (Genesee, 2006; Genesee & Nicoladis, 2007; Hoff & Rumiche, 2012). (To be fair to the field, starting with the study of monolingual development was reasonable as an initial research strategy, and current research on bilingual development stands firmly on the shoulders of the preceding decades of research on monolingual development.) A more applied motive for the increased interest in research on bilingualism and bilingual development is the growing number of bilingual children in schools around the world and the attendant concern about their academic achievement. Bilingual children often (but, importantly, not always) hear a minority language at home and attend school in a different language, the language of the cultural majority. On average, children from language minority homes have lower levels of academic achievement than non-minority children, both in the United States and elsewhere (National Center for Education Statistics, 2006; Scheele *et al.*, 2010). Because language skills are widely thought to play a role in accounting for what is termed the achievement gap between language minority and monolingual children, understanding the language skills of children from language minority homes is of concern to policy makers in many countries (Hoff, 2013; Oller & Eilers, 2002). As the number of bilingual children grows, the need for educational and clinical assessment of bilinguals also grows.

In sum, the expanding field of research on bilingual development and the increasing numbers of bilingual children in schools and clinical caseloads creates an urgent need for ways of assessing bilingual children. Together, the chapters in these books move the field towards meeting that need, laying out major issues and proposing solutions. This concluding commentary reviews some of the issues raised in these chapters and tries to add to the discussion.

Establishing Language Norms for Bilingual Children

One major issue in the assessment of bilingual children is the establishment or selection of norms against which the individual bilingual child is be evaluated. As Gathercole (2013) points out in the introductory chapter to *Issues in the Assessment of Bilinguals*, assessment typically requires comparing a child's performance to expectations, and those expectations are 'determined by our knowledge of *how similar children ... at similar stages of development have been able to perform*' (Gathercole, 2013: 3). In order to define expectations for the bilingual child (in testing parlance, to establish norms), we need to know what normal bilingual development looks like. Many chapters in these books remind us of Grosjean's oft-cited dictum that the bilingual is not two monolinguals in one (e.g. Grosjean, 1989). Although bilingual children – especially bilingual children who are dominant in the language of the test – often perform within the normal range of variation for monolingual children, it is still the case that the development of each language in bilingual children is affected by their dual language exposure (Hoff *et al.*, 2012). We see in multiple chapters in these volumes some of the ways in which bilingualism influences language development and performance in language testing. Children who are acquiring two languages initially develop each at a slower rate than the rate of language development in monolingual children (Gathercole, 2013). Failure to take this into account contributes to the over-identification of bilingual children as language impaired (Bedore *et al.*,

2005). Chapters in these volumes also show ways in which the course of development of each language is much like the course of typical development for monolingual children and not drastically altered by cross-linguistic influence (Abugov & Ravid, 2013; Gathercole *et al.*, 2013; see also Conboy & Thal, 2006; Marchman *et al.*, 2004). There is other evidence, however, that the rate of development in some domains of language knowledge is more affected by bilingualism than others, yielding what have been termed 'profile effects' in bilingual development (Oller *et al.*, 2007).

Norms for bilinguals need to take account not only of the fact that bilingual knowledge is different but also that bilingualism affects how children perform on tests of their knowledge. Bilinguals use their knowledge of one language to figure out the meaning of words and text in their other language (Genesee *et al.*, this volume; Stadthagen-González *et al.*, this volume). This makes expectations for performance not only different for monolinguals and bilinguals, but also different for bilinguals who know different language pairs, and different for bilinguals at different ages because the usefulness of cognate knowledge will depend on the relatedness of a bilingual's two languages and also, perhaps, on developmental level. For example, it seems to this minimally proficient reader of Spanish that there are proportionately more Spanish–English cognates in a scientific article than in a child's book.

Bilinguals need multiple norms. These chapters make it clear that expectations for bilingual children must differ depending on the circumstances of their bilingualism, and the circumstances of bilingual development vary widely on multiple dimensions. The amount of exposure to each language the bilingual individual experiences, the sources of children's exposure to each language, the age at which dual language exposure begins and the use of a minority language in the larger community outside the home are all factors that influence bilingual development and must be taken account of in forming expectations (e.g. Pérez-Tattam *et al.*, 2013; Place & Hoff, 2011; Thomas *et al.*, this volume). Some of the projects described in these books have begun to develop norms specific to different types of bilingual experience (e.g. Gathercole *et al.*, 2013; Peña *et al.*, this volume). Socio-economic status (SES) has a robust and substantial effect on language development (Hoff, 2006), and that also must be taken into account in the evaluation of the bilingual child. Many bilingual children are also children from low SES households, and thus their language skills reflect both influences. There is also variability within bilingual populations in SES; thus the expectations for all bilingual children should not be the same. And, SES is a source of variability between bilingual populations as well, making cross-population inferences difficult. For example, SES differences between populations may be the explanation of why the L2 skills of English–Hebrew children in Israel resemble those of monolingual Hebrew-speaking children more than the L2 skills of Turkish-English bilingual children in London resemble those of monolingual English-speaking children (Chiat *et al.*, 2013).

Cultural differences in norms of language use and familiarity with test taking also need to be taken into account in the assessment of bilingual children whose home culture may differ from the culture of the school, from the cultural background assumed by the materials or from the culture of assessment itself (e.g. Genesee *et al.*, this volume). Because so many factors shape bilingual development and the test performance of bilingual children, assessment of bilingual children must entail more than assessment of the skills under investigation. It must also include collecting information about the children's past and current opportunities to acquire those skills (Genesee *et al.*, this volume).

Expectations based on children with similar experiences are particularly important for the clinical purpose of identifying language impairment. As Peña *et al.* (this volume) point out, although we measure language *proficiency* for many purposes, the clinician is interested in measuring language *ability*, defined as the capacity for learning. Comparison to norms is the means of inferring ability from measures of proficiency. For other purposes, a comparison to norms may not be the point. The relevant expectations may be those of the curriculum. If instructional materials require a certain level of vocabulary and grammatical development, then it is important to know when a child does not meet those expectations – even if the cause of the child's language level is simply lack of language experience (Chiat *et al.*, 2013).

Identifying Measures and Procedures for Assessment

The assessment challenge arising from the influence of the multiple factors on bilingual development has prompted some to seek measures or procedures that are valid across differences in these many sources of variance.

Assessing both languages of the bilingual child

Many chapters emphasize the need to assess both languages in a bilingual child in order to adequately assess what the child knows. This, of course, requires assessment instruments for both languages. Some of the chapters in this book describe the development of instruments where few to none have existed before – for Basque (Ezeizabarrena *et al.*, this volume), for Irish (O'Toole, this volume), and for Cypriot Greek (Kambanaros & Grohmann, this volume).

Where instruments for both languages are available, the question arises of what one does with the results of assessment in two languages – again, what are the expectations for bilingual children? This is a topic with something of a history in the field of bilingualism. With respect to the assessment of early vocabulary – up to 30 months and using parent-report inventories – two different measures have been suggested: Total Vocabulary, which is the sum of the children's vocabulary (or raw vocabulary score) on both languages, and Conceptual Vocabulary. Conceptual Vocabulary is a measure of the number of concepts the child has a word for, and it is measured from language inventories by subtracting the number of items for which the child has a word in both languages from Total Vocabulary score. The Irish–English inventory described in this volume yields both a total and conceptual vocabulary score (O'Toole, this volume). There is evidence that at least for children up to 30 months, assessed with the MacArthur inventories, bilingual children's Total Vocabulary scores are very similar to the single-language vocabulary scores of SES-matched monolingual children (Hoff et al., 2012). Eventually bilinguals must have larger total vocabularies than monolinguals, because they know two languages to the monolingual's one. More research is needed to identify the point at which that bilingual advantage begins.

Another means of assessing conceptual vocabulary or using conceptual assessment to gauge language knowledge across a bilingual child's two languages is to use an administration procedure in which the child is tested in his or her dominant language and then asked for a response in the non-dominant language only where the child cannot respond in the language of testing. For example, the manual for the bilingual form of the *Expressive One Word Picture Vocabulary Test (EOWPVT)* instructs the examiner to identify the bilingual child's dominant language and ask the child to label each picture in that language (Brownell, 2000). Only if the child cannot provide a label is the child asked for it in his or her non-dominant language. This procedure yields a measure of the total number of pictures in the test for which the child has a word in at least one language, and that may be a valuable measure for identifying children with cognitive or language impairment. Whether conceptual measures are the best indicator of bilingual children's language development is a matter of some debate (Core et al., under review) and may depend on the purpose to which the assessment is being put (Barrueco et al., 2012). Certainly, conceptual assessment approaches do not yield measures of children's levels of development in their non-dominant language. And a testing approach such as that prescribed for the *EOWPVT* does not yield a measure of children's skill in either language alone (Barrueco et al., 2012).

Another procedural issue that arises in assessing two languages in bilingual children is who is to do the assessment. For caregiver reports, the same person can provide reports on both languages if the reporter is sufficiently proficient in both languages and in a position to know the child's proficiency in both languages. This is the procedure built into the inventory for Irish–English bilinguals (O'Toole, this volume, and has been done for Welsh–English bilinguals). In the assessment of young Spanish–English bilinguals using MacArthur inventories, separate report forms are used for each language, but frequently the same bilingual caregiver completes both the Spanish and English inventories. Data collected in this manner have shown high correlations with language measures based on spontaneous speech (Marchman & Martinez-Sussmann, 2002) and with measures of language exposure (Hoff et al., 2012; Place & Hoff, 2011). Combining reports from multiple caregivers can also be used. Using teacher report has been tried, but teachers seem to not be aware of their pupils' full vocabulary and to provide underestimates (Vagh et al., 2009). When standardized assessments are administered by professionals or researchers to older children, the question is whether to use the same bilingual examiner for both language assessments or to use different examiners, with each pretending to be or really being monolingual. Using two examiners can be logistically difficult and introduces a new source of variance in children's performance. However, when a single bilingual examiner is used, children may code switch and that complicates assessment of the children's skill levels in each language, considered separately (Hoff & Rumiche, 2012).

Identifying experience-free and culture-free measures

An alternative approach to finding meaningful measures of bilingual children's language knowledge is to try to tap deeper. The aim is to find tasks and measures that are less susceptible to contamination from social and cultural influences on bilingual children's test performance. The proposals here include measuring semantic development in each language (including indicators of fluency, understanding word relations and making word associations), measuring accuracy of sentence imitation as a gauge of morphosyntax (Chiat et al., 2013), and using processing measures as indicators of the 'quality' of lexical representations (Pérez et al., 2013). Pérez et al. show that reaction time measures may be sensitive to differences in language knowledge where vocabulary counts are not, a finding consistent with the evidence from very young children that those with larger vocabularies (and more language experience) are faster at processing the words they know than those with smaller vocabularies (and less language experience) and that bilingual children are faster at processing words in the language they hear more frequently (Fernald et al., 2006; Marchman et al., 2010).

When the purpose of assessment is to identify children with language impairment, the aim for assessment is to identify skills that are not susceptible to the influence of vagaries in bilingual children's experience and that distinguish typically developing from language impaired children (Letts, this volume; Peña et al., this volume). That is, the aim is to find a 'pure' measure of language learning ability. At one time non-word repetition was thought to be such a task. However, as the findings in these chapters and elsewhere show, children's task performance is always related to their exposure to the language in which the task is administered (Chiat et al., 2013; Parra et al., 2011). The distinction that Peña et al. (this volume) draw, between language *proficiency* and language *ability*, is crucial to the definition of language impairment, but there is no experience-free test of language ability. There is no way around using language proficiency as an indicator of language ability, and thus no way around the need for establishing expectations.

Identifying Equivalent Measures

Equivalency across languages

Many purposes require the assessment of one or both of a bilingual child's languages independent of knowledge in the other. An educator who needs to know if a child is ready to read certain English-language material might want an assessment of the child's English vocabulary, not his combined vocabulary. A researcher who wants to investigate factors that influence Spanish and English language development (or any other combination of languages) needs separate assessments of Spanish and English knowledge. When research and clinical reports describe a child as dominant in English or dominant in Spanish, the implication is that the child knows more in one language than in the other. For such a statement to be meaningful and supportable, the child's knowledge in each language must be assessed with instruments that yield measures that mean the same thing for each language.

There are many ways, some trivial and some profound, in which measures of language knowledge can fail to mean the same thing in two different languages. Lexical items are necessarily different – not just different phonological forms, but the word meanings and grammatical structures differ. As Ezeizabarrena and colleagues describe in their report of adapting the MacArthur–Bates CDI for Basque (Ezeizabarrena *et al.*, this volume), the items differ because children growing up in Basque-speaking regions don't talk about 'cowboys', but they do talk about 'ghosts'. And of course, the items pertaining to morphology and syntax are different from and wider ranging than those in English, because Basque is grammatically different and morphologically richer. This lack of equivalence is not unique to Basque and English. The Spanish version of the CDI has 125 (out of 680) lexical items not on the English version (e.g. *pollito* [chick], *mosca* [fly], *quesadilla, sandía* [watermelon], *perder* [to lose], *saber* [to know], *cenar* [to eat dinner], *así* [like this], *entre* [between], *enfrente* [in front of]), and the English version has 128 items with no equivalent on the Spanish version (e.g. *kitty, moose, cheerios, noodles, clap, lick, pour, about, around, off*). The grammatical complexity items differ between the Spanish and English forms as well where the languages have structures that are not equivalent.

The problem of cross-linguistic equivalency is not unique to the CDI and its adaptations. A widely used measure in the United States, *The Preschool*

Language Scale (Zimmerman *et al.*, 2002), has an English and a Spanish version that are very, but not completely, comparable. In the 4th edition, for example, one of the categories at the 2;6–2;11 level in the Spanish version is 'understands several pronouns (*me, mi, tú, tu*)'. There is no clear counterpart to this in English. Another problem, perhaps related to the need for noncomparable items across languages, is that the items that are the same (on their face, if not psychometrically) are at different age levels on different versions. For example, items that are designed to tap children's ability to understand expressions of part/whole relationships (e.g. *the door of the car*) are in the 2;6–2;11 group on the English version of the PLS-4, but their equivalents (e.g. *la puerta del carro*) are in the 3;0–3;11 category on the Spanish version. This difference can have large effects because the testing procedure calls for stopping the test once the child misses a certain number of items in a row. Thus, a bilingual child who does not know the pronoun system in Spanish would not ever be tested on part/whole relationships in Spanish, but that same child might be tested on part/whole relationships in English. A comparison of the child's ability to express part/whole relationships in English and Spanish could never be made. Another example of a difference between counterpart forms (which does not reflect intrinsic differences between the languages) occurs between the most current versions of the *Peabody Picture Vocabulary Test (PPVT)* and its Spanish counterpart, *Test de Vocabulario en Imágenes Peabody (TVIP)*, which were available in 2011 (Dunn & Dunn, 2007; Dunn *et al.*, 1986). The PPVT picture plates are large, detailed and in color. The TVIP picture plates are smaller, have less detail and are in black and white.

Even where procedures and measures seem comparable, differences between the languages could produce differences in the meaning of a language score. For example, it appears that acquiring a 50-word vocabulary is a greater accomplishment for children acquiring Danish than it is for children acquiring many other languages, as evidenced by the fact that this milestone is typically reached at a later age among Danish children (Bleses *et al.*, 2008). The reason seems to be that Danish has a very high vowel-to-consonant ratio, making identifying word boundaries difficult. This causes difficulty for children first breaking into the language system, but the difficulty does not persist. Thus, the extent to which a vocabulary count means something different for a child acquiring English and Danish changes with development.

The difficulties of achieving comparability with respect to grammar can only be greater than for vocabulary, as languages differ in the devices they use (e.g. word order or grammatical morphology) – both overall and to serve specific functions. Gathercole and colleagues' approach in developing tests for Welsh and English is to create tests of structures that are comparable in the sense of performing the same function (e.g. marking negation, marking past tense), although not necessarily using the same device (Gathercole *et al.*,

2013). This allows comparison of what a child can do in each language and, for some purposes, this may be the most relevant assessment metric. For research purposes, however, the requirements are greater and the difficulties of meeting those requirements are also greater. If, for example, one wanted to ask whether the function relating home input to grammatical development is different for Welsh and English, one would need more directly comparable measures of grammatical development in each language. As Peña et al. (this volume) point out, linguistic equivalence and psychometric equivalence are not the same thing.

Norm-referenced scores appear at first blush to be a solution to the incommensurability across languages of direct measures of knowledge. Percentile or standard scores provide indices of children's progress in each language on the same numerical scale. However, norm-referenced scores have another source of non-equivalency. The reference groups used in the standardization for each language can and sometimes clearly do differ. For example, in the norming group for the English CDI, 8% of mothers had less than a high school education while in the norming group for the Spanish IDHC, 30% of the mothers had less than a high school education (Fenson et al., 2007; Jackson-Maldonado et al., 2003). As a result, a 30-month-old child who knows 616 words on the English version (the CDI) is at the 65th percentile among monolingual English children, while a child who knows 616 words on the Spanish version (the IDHC) is at the 80th percentile according to the Spanish monolingual norms. A bilingual child who knows the same number of words in English and in Spanish will look Spanish dominant, if norm-referenced scores are used.

Equivalency across ages and domains

In order to plot an individual child's progress or to conduct longitudinal studies, one also needs measurement invariance across time (Hofer et al., 2012). Children at different ages have different metalinguistic and test-taking skills, and that can complicate the development of procedures to use with children of different ages (Unsworth & Blom, 2010). A more profoundly difficult problem is that the nature of children's linguistic knowledge changes with development. Language development is not the sort of thing that can be easily measured in the same units from birth to maturity.

The issue of measurement equivalence also arises when one wishes to make comparisons across domains of language development. For example, research might ask whether lexical development is more affected by bilingualism than grammatical development. Clinicians might ask whether a particular child is more delayed in one domain or another. To do this properly, one needs measures in each domain that are equally sensitive to developmental change, and that can be difficult to achieve (Dixon & Marchman, 2007).

Equivalency across monolingual and bilingual populations

Often the purpose of language assessment is to predict an individual's future probability of success at some academic endeavor and to make an assignment or admission decision on that basis. Use of the same assessment instrument and criterion scores for monolingual and bilingual children or adults assumes the same relation between predictor and criterion in both populations. That is not necessarily the case. For example, elementary-school bilingual children have been found to perform better in verbal memory tasks than their single-language vocabulary size would predict, even though vocabulary is a predictor of task performance in both monolinguals and bilinguals (Bialystok & Feng, 2011), and bilingual students in college have been found to have higher grade point averages than their SAT scores would predict, although SAT scores predict grade point in both monolinguals and bilinguals (Pearson, 1993).

Bilingual Assessment in Educational Settings

The assessment of bilingual children for educational purposes entails particular challenges. Not only oral language skills but particularly literacy skills are the target of education and thus of assessment. All the issues that apply to assessing oral language apply also to assessing bilingual children's reading and writing skills in two languages. Although the focus of most classrooms and curricula is often on developing skills in the majority language, knowing children's skill levels in both their languages is relevant for the assessment of children's abilities and for educational planning. The child who reads well in Spanish but poorly in English has different needs from the child who does not read at all. There is the challenge of identifying the source of difficulties that bilingual children may experience. In evaluating bilingual children's literacy skills in their second language, it can be difficult to distinguish reading difficulty arising from reading impairment from reading difficulty arising from incomplete acquisition of the target language (Genesee et al., this volume). There is also the question of what components of language skill should be measured for maximum predictive value (Genesee et al., this volume).

Particularly for literacy, a question with broad practical implication is whether language or literacy skills in one language predict the acquisition of literacy in another language. As Genesee and colleagues remind us, the validity of the answer we get depends on having accurately measured the right things at the right level of granularity. In interpreting the research on predictors of children's language and literacy, it is important to remember that a null result may mean only that the measures did not adequately capture the relevant individual differences in the underlying construct. Furthermore, like oral language skills, literacy has multiple components. Writing can be assessed with respect to both form and content (Rodríguez-González, this volume); reading, Genesee *et al.*'s results show, must be assessed in terms of both word-level and text-level skills. Children's perceptions of their language and literacy skills are also important targets of assessment (Rodríguez-González, this volume).

'Assessment is an essential part of the teaching process' (Cenoz *et al.*, 2013). Assessing the knowledge children bring with them to the classroom is necessary for selecting instructional materials (Burns, 2013) and assessment of what children are learning through instruction is necessary for program evaluation. Although evaluating educational outcomes is difficult, contentious, subject to misuse and highly politicized (Caldas, 2013), it is still the case that parents, policy makers, voters and other stakeholders in education have a right to assessments of the effects of the educational programs they support.

Conclusions

The chapters in these books shed new light on the nature of bilingual development and bilingual knowledge, and in doing so they highlight the close relation between the theoretical enterprise of understanding the process of language acquisition and the practical enterprise of devising means to assess what children have acquired. Every assessment of language and literacy entails a theory of what constitutes language and literacy skill. Every finding that measures of children's language skill reflect their language exposure has the theoretical implication that there is nothing in language development that manifests itself without requiring language experience and the practical implication that there will be no language-general diagnostic indicator of language impairment. The complex and varied nature of the circumstances that give rise to bilingualism and create variability in patterns of bilingual skill reveal the larger truth that language acquisition is paced and shaped by the cultural, societal and family context in which it occurs. Because of the complexity of bilingual outcomes and the circumstances that shape them, a recurring theme in this volume is the urging of caution in the assessment of bilingual children.

The work described in these volumes brings the field closer to being able to accurately assess the language knowledge of children and adults whose language knowledge encompasses more than one language and whose language learning experiences vary in multiple dimensions. These chapters make clear that many issues remain to be solved, as they also advance the conversations the field must have to move forward in developing instruments and procedures that address these issues.

References

Abugov, N. and Ravid, D. (2013) Assessing Yiddish plurals in acquisition: Impacts of bilingualism. In V.C.M. Gathercole (ed.) *Issues in the Assessment of Bilinguals* (pp. 90–110). Bristol: Multilingual Matters.

Barrueco, S., López, M., Ong, C. and Lozano, P. (2012) *Assessing Spanish-English Bilingual Preschoolers: A Guide to Best Approaches and Measures*. Baltimore, MD: Brookes Publishing.

Bedore, L.M., Peña, E.D., García, M. and Cortez, C. (2005) Clinical forum: Conceptual versus monolingual scoring: When does it make a difference? *Language, Speech, and Hearing Services in Schools* 36 (3), 188–200; doi: 10.1044/0161-1461(2005/020).

Bialystok, E. and Feng, X. (2011) Language proficiency and its implications for monolingual and bilingual children. In A.Y. Durgunoğlu and C. Goldenberg (eds) *Dual-language Learners: The Development and Assessment of Oral and Written Language*. New York: Guildford Press.

Bleses, D., Vach, W., Slott, M., Wehberg, S., Thomsen, P., Madsen, T.O. and Basbøll, H. (2008) Early vocabulary development in Danish and other languages: A CDI-based comparison. *Journal of Child Language* 35, 619–650.

Brownell, R. (ed.) (2000) *Expressive One-word Vocabulary Test* (3rd edn). Novato, CA: Academic Therapy.

Burns, R. (2013) Assessment and instruction in multilingual classrooms. In V.C.M. Gathercole (ed.) *Issues in the Assessment of Bilinguals* (pp. 162–185). Bristol: Multilingual Matters.

Caldas, S. (2013) Assessment of academic performance: The impact of No Child Left Behind policies on bilingual education: A ten year retrospective. In V.C.M. Gathercole (ed.) *Issues in the Assessment of Bilinguals* (pp. 205–231). Bristol: Multilingual Matters.

Cenoz, J., Arozena, E. and Gorter, D. (2013) Assessing multilingual students' writing skills in Basque, Spanish and English. In V.C.M. Gathercole (ed.) *Issues in the Assessment of Bilinguals* (pp. 186–205). Bristol: Multilingual Matters.

Chiat, S., Armon-Lotem, S., Marinis, T., Polišenská, K., Roy, P. and Seeff-Gabriel, B. (2013) Assessment of language abilities in sequential bilingual children: The potential of sentence imitation tasks. In V.C.M. Gathercole (ed.) *Issues in the Assessment of Bilinguals* (pp. 56–89). Bristol: Multilingual Matters.

Conboy, B.T. and Thal, D.J. (2006) Ties between the lexicon and grammar: Cross-sectional and longitudinal studies of bilingual toddlers. *Child Development* 77, 712–735.

Dixon, J.A. and Marchman, V.A. (2007) Grammar and the lexicon: Developmental ordering in language acquisition. *Child Development* 78, 190–212.

Dunn, L.M. and Dunn, D.M. (2007) *Peabody Picture Vocabulary Test* (4th edn). Minneapolis, MN: NCS Pearson.

Dunn, L.M., Padilla, E.R., Lugo, D.E. and Dunn, L.M. (1986) *Test de vocabulario en imágenes Peabody*. Minneapolis, MN: NCS Pearson.

Fenson, L., Marchman, V.A., Thal, D.J., Dale, P.S., Reznick, J.S. and Bates, E. (2007) *MacArthur-bates Communicative Development Inventories: User's Guide and Technical Manual* (2nd edn). Baltimore, MD: Paul H. Brookes Publishing Company.

Fernald, A. and Marchman, V.A. (2011) Causes and consequences of variability in early language learning. In I. Arnon and E.V. Clark (eds) *Experience, Variation and Generalization: Learning a First Language* (pp. 181–202). Amsterdam: John Benjamins.

Fernald, A., Perfors, A. and Marchman, V.A. (2006) Picking up speed in understanding: Speech processing efficiency and vocabulary growth across the second year. *Developmental Psychology* 42, 98–116.

Gathercole, V.C.M. (2013) Assessment of multi-tasking wonders: Music, Olympics, and language. In V.C.M. Gathercole (ed.) *Issues in the Assessment of Bilinguals* (pp. 1–19). Bristol: Multilingual Matters.

Gathercole, V.C.M., Thomas, E.M., Roberts, E., Hughes, C. and Hughes, E.K. (2013) Why assessment needs to take exposure into account: Vocabulary and grammatical abilities in bilingual children. In V.C.M. Gathercole (ed.) *Issues in the Assessment of Bilinguals* (pp. 20–55). Bristol: Multilingual Matters.

Genesee, F. (2006) Bilingual first language acquisition in perspective. In P. McCardle and E. Hoff (eds) *Childhood Bilingualism: Research on Infancy Through School Age* (pp. 45–67). Clevedon: Multilingual Matters.

Genesee, F. and Nicoladis, E. (2007) Bilingual first language acquisition. In E. Hoff and M. Shatz (eds) *Blackwell Handbook of Language Development* (pp. 324–342). Chichester: Wiley-Blackwell.

Grosjean, F. (1989) Neurolinguists, beware! The bilingual is not two monolinguals in one person. *Brain and Language* 36, 3–15.

Hofer, S.M., Thorvaldsson, V. and Piccinin, A.M. (2012) Foundational issues of design and measurement in developmental research. In B. Laursen, T.D. Little and N.A. Card (eds) *Handbook of Developmental Research Methods* (pp. 3–16). New York: Guildford Press.

Hoff, E. (2006) How social contexts support and shape language development. *Developmental Review* 26, 55–88.

Hoff, E. (2013) Interpreting the early language trajectories of children from low SES and language minority homes: Implications for closing achievement gaps. *Developmental Psychology* 49, 4–14.

Hoff, E., Core, C., Place, S., Rumiche, R., Señor, M. and Parra, M. (2012) Dual language exposure and early bilingual development. *Journal of Child Language* 39, 1–27.

Hoff, E. and Rumiche, R. (2012) Studying children in bilingual environments. In E. Hoff (ed.) *Research Methods in Child Language: A Practical Guide*. Boston, MA: Wiley/Blackwell.

Jackson-Maldonado, D., Thal, D.J., Fenson, L., Marchman, V., Newton, T. and Conboy, B. (2003) *El inventario del desarrollo de habilidades comunicativas: User's Guide and Technical Manual*. Baltimore, MD: Brookes Publishing.

Marchman, V.A., Fernald, A. and Hurtado, N. (2010) How vocabulary size in two languages relates to efficiency in spoken word recognition by young Spanish–English bilinguals. *Journal of Child Language* 37, 817–840.

Marchman, V.A. and Martínez-Sussmann, D. (2002) Concurrent validity of caregiver/parent report measure of language for children who are learning both English and Spanish. *Journal of Speech, Language, and Hearing Research* 45, 983–997.

Marchman, V.A., Martínez-Sussmann, C. and Dale, P.S. (2004) The language-specific nature of grammatical development: Evidence from bilingual language learners. *Developmental Science* 7, 212–224.

National Center for Educational Statistics (2006) *The Condition of Education*. Washington, DC: US Department of Education.

Oller, D.K. and Eilers, R. (eds) (2002) *Language and Literacy in Bilingual Children*. Clevedon: Multilingual Matters.

Oller, D.K., Pearson, B.Z. and Cobo-Lewis, A.B. (2007) Profile effects in early bilingual language and literacy. *Applied Psycholinguistics* 28 (2), 191–230.

Parra, M., Hoff, E. and Core, C. (2011) Relations among language exposure, phonological memory, and language development in Spanish–English bilingually-developing two-year-olds. *Journal of Experimental Child Psychology* 108, 113–125.

Pearson, B.Z. (1993) Predictive validity of the scholastic aptitude test (SAT) for Hispanic bilingual students. *Hispanic Journal of Behavioral Sciences* 15, 342–356.

Pearson, B.Z., Fernandez, S.C. and Oller, D.K. (1995) Cross-language synonyms in the lexicons of bilingual infants: One language or two? *Journal of Child Language* 22, 345–368.

Pérez, M. A., Izura, C., Stadthagen-González, H. and Marín, J. (2013) Assessment of bilinguals' performance in lexical tasks using reaction times. In V.C.M. Gathercole (ed.) *Issues in the Assessment of Bilinguals* (pp. 130–161). Bristol: Multilingual Matters.

Pérez-Tattam, R., Gathercole, V.C.M., Yavas, F. and Stadthagen-González, H. (2013) Measuring grammatical knowledge and abilities in bilinguals: Implications for assessment and testing. In V.C.M. Gathercole (ed.) *Issues in the Assessment of Bilinguals* (pp. 111–129). Bristol: Multilingual Matters.
Place, S. and Hoff, E. (2011) Properties of dual language exposure that influence two-year-olds' bilingual proficiency. *Child Development* 82, 1834–1849.
Scheele, A.F., Leseman, P.P.M. and Mayo, A.Y. (2010) The home language environment of monolingual and bilingual children and their language proficiency. *Applied Psycholinguistics* 31, 117–140.
Unsworth, S. and Blom, E. (2010) Comparing L1 children, L2 children and L2 adults. In E. Blom and S. Unsworth (eds) *Experimental Methods in Language Acquisition Research* (pp. 201–222). Amsterdam: John Benjamins.
Vagh, S.B., Pan, B.A. and Mancilla-Martinez, J. (2009) Measuring growth in bilingual and monolingual children's English productive vocabulary development: The utility of combining parent and teacher report. *Child Development* 80, 1545–1563.
Zimmerman, I.L., Steiner, V.G. and Pond, R.E. (2002) *Preschool Language Scale* (4th edn). San Antonio, TX: Harcourt Assessment, The Psychological Corporation.

Index of Tests and Measures

Index of Languages

Index of Terms